Praise for *Beyond Antibiotics:*

"Excellent book. Conclusions are discussed in detail in a clear and easy-to-read manner. But, even better, is the description of how we can recognize common ailments, their origins, and what we can do about them."—**Abram Hoffer, M.D., Ph.D.,** author of *Orthomolecular Nutrition*

"*Beyond Antibiotics* sends a clarion warning to the consumer—change your microflora at your own peril! Chemical solutions to problems of internal balance are always risky—and Drs. Schmidt, Sehnert, and Smith amply document the dangers of overuse of antibiotics."
—**Marc Lappé, Ph.D.,** author of *When Antibiotics Fail*

"*Beyond Antibiotics* contains much valuable information—unknown to most regular physicians—about how to protect immunity and how to treat common infectious illnesses without using prescription antibiotics. The authors maintain a balance between conventional and alternative medicine, always emphasizing the importance of self-care."
—**Andrew Weil, M.D.,** author of *Health and Healing* and *Natural Health, Natural Medicine*

"It is excellent to see such a comprehensive approach to patient care by experienced physicians who are interested in helping their patients as much as possible without having to resort to potentially toxic pharmaceutical preparations, while suggesting effective drug treatment when there is no obvious nutritional alternative."
—**Dr. Stephen Davies,** author of *Nutritional Medicine*

"The scope of this book reflects the new and better trend in 20th century medical care. More and more informed adults realize that the best answer for children and adults is to find out exactly why they are ill and try to eliminate the cause. This is particularly true if antibiotics are repeatedly required to treat recurrent infections.

"This book gives a balanced review of explanations and choices. It shows fast, simple, inexpensive, and practical answers that should help some individuals to feel better on a long-term basis. It provides valuable insight to help them understand why they are ill and, more important, what they, as individuals, can do to improve their situations.

"I can hardly wait to see this book in print. I will definitely recommend it for my allergic and environmentally-ill patients—so many are sensitive to antibiotics, or to the dyes, sugar, corn, and artificial flavors used in many drugs."
—**Doris J. Rapp, M.D.,** Environmental Allergy Center, author of *Is This Your Child?*

Beyond Antibiotics

Healthier Options for Families

Dr. Michael A. Schmidt

Dr. Lendon H. Smith

Dr. Keith W. Sehnert

North Atlantic Books
Berkeley, California

Beyond Antibiotics: Healthier Options for Families

Copyright © 1993 by Dr. Michael A. Schmidt

ISBN 1-55643-134-X
All rights reserved

Published by
North Atlantic Books
2800 Woolsey Street
Berkeley, California 94705

Cover and book design by Paula Morrison
Typeset by Patricia McGillis
Printed in the United States of America

Beyond Antibiotics: Healthier Options for Families is sponsored by the Society for the Study of Native Arts and Sciences, a nonprofit educational corporation whose goals are to develop an educational and cross-cultural perspective linking various scientific, social, and artistic fields; to nurture a holistic view of arts, sciences, humanities, and healing; and to publish and distribute literature on the relationship of mind, body, and nature.

Dedicated to the spirit of holism
in medicine and to all those who strive
to bring about meaningful change.

Acknowledgements

We would like to thank the many physicians, healers, researchers and educators whose ideas and concepts appear in this book. As with any area of human endeavor, the work of our predecessors and peers is vital to the advancement and illumination of new ideas.

There are numerous friends and colleagues who have contributed ideas and insights that have helped make this book what it is. To them we are grateful: Russell M. Jaffe, M.D., Ph.D., Jeffrey S. Bland, Ph.D., William G. Crook, M.D., Sidney Wolfe, M.D., Leo Galland, M.D., Jonathan Wright, M.D., Paul Westby, D.C., Emanuel Cheraskin, M.D., D.M.D., Abram Hoffer, M.D., Ph.D., Kurt Schnaubelt, Ph.D., Alan Gaby, M.D., Linus Pauling, Ph.D., Doris Rapp, M.D., Sherry Rogers, M.D., Marc Lappé, Ph.D., Dana Ullman, M.P.H. and Stephen Davies, M.D. These individuals are among the leaders in the field of preventive medicine.

We are also grateful for the work of Martin Seligman, Ph.D., Larry Dossey, M.D., George Solomon, M.D., Robert Ornstein, Ph.D., David Sobel, M.D., Stephen Locke, M.D., Jean Achterberg, Ph.D. and others for their exciting and pioneering work in the field of brain/mind/body and psychoneuroimmunology.

We would also like to thank the *Milbank Memorial Fund Quarterly* for permission to reprint material that appears in Chapter 2 of this book. A special thanks also to The National Geographic Society.

We are grateful to Kathy Glass and Paula Morrison who put their editorial and artistic touches on this book. Their efforts have helped give clarity and consistency to what began as a mountain of paper.

We owe a special debt of gratitude to our wives who continue to offer their patience, understanding and insight to the work we do. They seem always willing to endure our humorous ways as well as our sometimes intense intellectual gymnastics.

Finally, we are indebted to our patients, who have been the greatest teachers of all. They have taught us compassion, understanding and a true wisdom that is gained only from the world of experience.

A Note to Readers

We have written this book to serve as a general reference for those concerned about the use of antibiotics and ways to reduce the chance of infections. While we have made some basic recommendations about health and illness, we cannot accept medical or legal responsibility for having the contents of this book considered as a prescription for any person. Some of the guidelines outlined in this book are based on time-honored, common sense approaches that anyone can safely use. However, before undertaking any specific recommendations outlined in this book, it would be wise to consult with your doctor. You and your physician or licensed health care professional must take full responsibility for the uses made of this book.

Table of Contents

Foreword, Dr. Michael A. Schmidt xv

Introduction, Dr. Lendon H. Smith xxi

Preface, Dr. Keith W. Sehnert xxv

Part I: Are Antibiotics the Best Medicine? 1

Chapter 1. Casualties of the War on Germs 3

   The War on Germs....................................... 5

   Ask the Right Questions 9

Chapter 2. Antibiotics: What Your Doctor May Not Tell You . 13

   The Paradoxes of Antibiotic Use 14

   Antibiotics and Infection: Not What You Think 15

   The Perils of Antibiotic Use 18

   Bugs, Drugs and Susceptibility........................ 30

   Science, Politics or Economics......................... 32

   Age- and Sex-Related Concerns 33

   In the Hospital 38

   At the Dentist 40

   Doctor and Patient Attitudes.......................... 42

   Public Perception: The Myths of Antibiotic Use 45

   But Doctor, Are You Sure?............................. 47

   Doctors Are Different 48

   Doctors Are Not Taught Alternatives in Medical School .. 51

   Are Antibiotics Being Overused in Your Care?........... 53

   Why Use Antibiotics?................................. 54

Part II: Why We Get Sick 59

Chapter 3. The Miracle of Immunity....................... 61

Chapter 4. Food, Nutrition and Infection Susceptibility....... 69

   How Nutrition Affects Immunity and Infection
     Susceptibility.. 69

How Infection Affects Nutritional Status. 72
Food Allergy, Intolerance and Immunity 74
Nutritional Deficiency: More Common Than You Think . . 80
What Affects Your Nutritional Needs?. 82
Excess Sugar and Fat Can Lower Immunity 83
The Importance of Fiber 85
Anti-Nutrients and Immunity. 87
The Eating Environment. 88
Food, Nutrition and Coping 89
Thyroid Problems and Altered Immunity 91
Infections *From* Your Food. 93
Eating for Optimum Immunity 94
Do You Need Vitamin and Mineral Supplements?. 96
Immune-Boosting Nutrients. 97
A Summary of Things to Do 103

Chapter 5. Environmental Threats to a Healthy
Immune System. 105
Environmental Illness. 107
Toxins Inside and Out. 107
Your Total Toxic Load 108
Toxins From Within. 109
Parasites Lurking About 110
Heavy Metals and Immunity 111
Dental Amalgams: A Threat to Immunity?. 113
The Electromagnetic Sea. 115
Are You Exposed to Toxic Substances? 117
Is Your Building Making You Sick? 118
Mold in the Home: Common Environmental Insult. 120
Air Pollution and Respiratory Infection. 120
Exposure on the Job 122
Pollutants Cause Malnourishment 123
A "Good Diet" is Not Enough 124
Signs of a Toxic Body 125

Reducing Toxins in Your Body 125
Testing for Toxic Exposure 126
The Low Temperature Sauna: Powerful Detoxifier 127
A Strategy for Living in Modern Times 128
A Summary of Things to Do 130
Chapter 6. Heredity and Lifestyle 131
Is it in Your Genes? 131
A Legacy for Our Children 135
Hygiene, Lifestyle and Personal Habits 136
A Summary of Things to Do 152
Chapter 7. Mood, Mind, Stress and Infections 155
Stress, Life Events & Infections 156
Stress and the Common Cold 160
Black Monday Syndrome 161
Stress and the Immune System 161
Negative Effects From Stress Are Not Inevitable 163
It's Not Always the Stress, But How We Cope 164
Power Coping and the Art of Letting Go 167
Are You an Optimist or Pessimist? Your Cells Know 168
Great Expectations 171
Abuse and Illness 172
Power and Self-Efficacy 172
Social Support and Meaningful Relationships 172
Anger, Cynicism and Hostility 174
The Power of Beliefs 176
Giving Mirth: Laughter May Be the Best Medicine 177
Illness as Metaphor 178
Don't Blame the Victim 179
Is There an Immune-Competent Personality? 180
A Summary of Things to Do 181

Part III: Natural Medicine 183
Chapter 8. Vitamin C: Powerful Preventive and Treatment . .185

Different Needs 186

On the Wrong Course. 188

Vitamin C and Infectious Disease. 188

Vitamin C in Action: What It Can Do. 192

The Right Dose. 193

Vitamin C and Animals 195

Deficiency Signs 195

Is Vitamin C Safe?. 196

The Vindication of Vitamin C 197

Basic Rules for Vitamin C Use 198

Chapter 9. Boosting Immunity Naturally: Complementary
Treatments Old and New. 201

Herbal Medicine: Is the Cure in the Jungle?. 202

Essential Plant Oils: A Medical Breakthrough
for Infection? 206

Homeopathy and Infection:
Stellar History, Brilliant Future 212

Hands-On Healing. 215

The Logical Step. 218

Part IV: Selfcare/Wellcare. 221

Chapter 10. Common Conditions for Which Antibiotics
Are Prescribed: What You Can Do 223

Acne. 225

Bladder Infection Cystitis) 226

Bronchitis. 229

The Common Cold 230

Earaches 232

Fever 235

Influenza (The Flu) 237

Intestinal Infection with Diarrhea 238

Post-Antibiotic Syndrome. 239

Rhinitis/Stuffy Nose 241

Sinusitis. 243

Teething in Children 245
Tonsillitis/Sore Throat 246
Vaginitis (Yeast Infection) 248
In General 250
Chapter 11. 50 (or so) Ways To Boost Immunity and Avoid
Antibiotics 251
Mood, Mind and Emotions 251
Lifestyle 253
Diet and Nutrition 255
Social 256
Spiritual 257
When You Feel Illness Approaching 258
Environment 258
Medicine Has Become Serious Business 259
Chapter 12. About the Healthier Options 261
Should You Say "No" When the Doctor Says "Yes"? 264
Your Health Care Team 265
The Cause of Illness 266
References 271
Index 297

Foreword

In March 1991, I appeared on a Miami radio program with two holistic physicians. The topic was how we manage and prevent infections using nutrition, botanical medicine and other means. The discussion eventually centered on the health of our own children. One doctor commented that of his five children between the ages of 3 and 13, none had ever been on antibiotics. The other doctor remarked that none of his five children between the ages of 3 and 11 had ever received antibiotics. I added that my then three-year-old son had also never been on antibiotics. Several weeks later, I spoke with a nurse who was the wife of a holistic physician. Of their nine children between the ages of 3 and 21, none had ever been treated with antibiotics.

This was astonishing. Was it possible that these children never got sick? Had they never suffered from bacterial (or viral) infections? What was the magic formula that allowed all these families to avoid antibiotic use while their friends and neighbors received the drugs for many common ailments? While generally very healthy, these children did experience bacterial and viral infections like all other children (although less frequent). However, rather than being treated with antibiotics, which kill germs but do nothing else for the child, they were treated with immune-building alternatives. The course of their illnesses were generally very short and recurrent infections were rare.

This was in stark contrast to the families of a group of family practice residents I was recently asked to speak to at a large Minneapolis hospital. The problem: their own children were constantly sick and were on antibiotics off-and-on for the better part of the winter. The children were sickly, coughing and had perpetual runny noses. These physicians wondered if there was any way they could improve the health of their children and get them off antibiotics. (The view changes when it hits close to home!) They were frustrated by the limitations of using antibiotics alone and hoped I might provide them with information on using diet, nutrition, herbs, acupressure and other ways of boosting immunity.

The differences between the families just described reflect a basic difference in philosophy. The holistic doctor views the patient as a whole and directs treatment to the patient during infection. The allopathic doctor typically views this type of illness as the result of bacterial invasion. Their treatment is directed toward the bacteria. We are of the former philosophy. We believe there are better ways to approach illness than the means being used by most allopathic doctors today.

The title of this book, *Beyond Antibiotics,* suggests that we must expand the sometimes nearsighted view of merely killing bacteria and look for the reasons we succumb to infection. We go beyond antibiotics by addressing these underlying factors.

The subtitle *Healthier Options for Families* implies that there are better approaches to many illnesses for which antibiotics are now given. The options are:

1. Use antibiotics alone. Although this is how antibiotics are traditionally used, it *is never* the healthier option because it does not:

   • Address the underlying reasons we become sick.

   • Address the side effects that can occur with antibiotic use.

   • Address the bodily effect of infection itself (eg. zinc and vitamin A loss).

2. Address the dietary, nutritional, psychological, social, lifestyle and other factors discussed in this book *in conjunction with* antibiotics. Used in this way, antibiotics may be the healthier option.

3. Address the factors discussed in this book, thereby eliminating the need for antibiotics. Sometimes, avoiding antibiotics is the healthier option.

4. Avoid becoming sick. This is perhaps the healthiest option. If one uses some basic strategies, common illnesses can be avoided or reduced. In this way, the use of antibiotics is avoided.

For example, pessimists suffer twice the number of infectious illnesses as optimists. If you are a pessimist, you might improve your health by becoming more of an optimist. Similarly, couch potatoes have more sluggish immune systems and experience more infections than those who exercise moderately. By simply increasing your level of physical activity, perhaps by walking 30 minutes daily, you might improve immunity and avoid the use of antibiotics. In this book, we discuss over 100 additional ways to boost immunity that may help you avoid the need for antibiotics.

This is not a book about disease, but a book about health. We are not urging you to treat diseases for that is the domain of doctors. Our goal is to empower you by giving you the means to enhance health, boost resistance to illness and use sound preventive strategies that will help you and your family avoid the use of antibiotics where possible.

The reader should recognize that the views expressed in this book do not represent the consensus opinion among allopathic doctors. Our views may, in fact, be considered heretical. However, the views expressed here are being shared by a growing number of physicians, researchers and public health officials who find it increasingly more difficult to overlook the emerging evidence. It is our hope that this book stirs debate and rouses both the public and medicine out of the complacency with which it has so long been afflicted regarding antibiotics and our resistance to infectious diseases.

I recognize that many physicians accustomed to using antibiotics as a first line of defense in treating illness will balk at the interpretation of the evidence presented in this book. Indeed, many will likely become irate at the notion that antibiotics are being misused to the extent we suggest. Yet, one cannot reject our thesis out-of-hand. The evidence is compelling, if not overwhelming, that we must take a new look at the current approach to the treatment of infectious illness and a new approach to the use of antibiotics.

We expect to be criticized for being against the use of antibiotics. This criticism will be undeserved for we are not against the *use* of antibiotics when the necessary diagnostic and therapeutic methods have been used. It is the *abuse* of antibiotics that we oppose. The evidence that we present that antibiotics are being abused and how is startling. Critics will also argue that to consider our advice would be to risk taking us back to the pre-antibiotic era when infectious diseases were rampant. The paradox in this argument is that the reverse may be true. Organisms associated with staph infections, gonorrhea and other diseases, once easily treated with antibiotics, are now resistant to almost all antibiotics typically used. According to Harvard professor and Nobel Laureate Walter Gilbert, "there may be a time down the road when 80 percent to 90 percent of infections will be resistant to all known antibiotics." A chilling thought!

We hope to avoid this by bringing about changes in the way antibiotics are used and by showing ways to boost immunity, thus reducing reliance upon antibiotics. In this book, we will show that changes in lifestyle, nutrition, diet, hygiene and other factors were largely responsible for the past decline in infectious disease—not antibiotics. These will be the tools used in the future. In addition, there have been many breakthroughs in the use of natural medicines to boost immunity.

In the final analysis, the important question remains, "Is it possible to care for illness without antibiotics, or at least reduce our reliance upon antibiotics?" To answer this, we can look at many scientific studies and also speak theoretically, but the real answer lies in whether anyone has done this in real life. In the beginning of this foreword, I spoke of four families, a total of 20 children who had never received antibiotics. In Chapter 6, we discuss a survey comparing the health of 200 pediatricians' children with that of the children of 200 holistic doctors. Nearly 50 percent of the children of these holistic doctors had never received antibiotics. This was in stark comparison to the pediatricians' children in whom less than 12 percent could say the same. Were the children in the former group merely fortunate? Perhaps, but such examples suggest that it is possible to minimize our use of these drugs.

What is the model used to accomplish this. What are the secrets? Can the principles be applied to the average family? The answer to the third question is "yes." The principles used by these families and holistic doctors are shared in this book. One of the most important factors, however, is that you become what Dr. Sehnert calls an "Activated Patient." This means that you agree to take charge of your own and your family's health. Do not surrender control of your health to doctors. Use your doctors for diagnosis and advice, and consider their recommendations thoughtfully. Become educated in basic methods of selfcare. Simply saying "no" to antibiotics, then doing nothing, is unwise. I, for one, am comforted by the knowledge that antibiotics exist, should I need them. The operative word is "need."

There is no guarantee that using the methods in this book will prevent you from getting infections, or that they will ensure that you will recover from an infection without using antibiotics. The information contained in this book has been taken from the medical literature, the clinical experience of different physicians worldwide and our clinical experiences. We can say that, in the past, people have been able to prevent infections and build immunity during infection without antibiotics by "wise" applications of methods similar to those discussed in this book.

Do not be a martyr. After reading this book you may decide that you will never use antibiotics again. The evidence for this viewpoint is compelling and tempts one to think this way. However, that would be foolish. Gather all the evidence you can. Question your doctors. Take charge of your health.

In *Beyond Antibiotics* we provide you with ways to find the *healthier options* for your family.

Michael A. Schmidt, B.S., D.C., C.C.N.
Anoka, MN
1992

Introduction

I am a consultant in the clinic at the National College of Naturopathic Medicine in Portland, Oregon. I have been acting as an observer and advisor while the junior and senior students work up patients. Many of the patients are there because they have been treated by allopathic methods and they have found them unacceptable. They are disappointed, sometimes disgusted, and frequently angry about the treatment they have received from their medical doctors.

Naturopathic medicine incorporates the use of vitamins, minerals, herbs, massage, hydrotherapy, homeopathy and other modalities. The students interview and examine patients and then present their findings to one of the naturopathic physicians who serve as clinic consultants. The students outline their treatment plan and then, with the doctor, they work out the best method of dealing with the problem. As a pediatrician, I am anxious to discover drugless ways to treat the conditions that were so common in my general practice.

Here is an example: A child was brought to the emergency clinic at the school on a Saturday with a cold, a fever of 101 degrees, pain, and a red hot, bulging ear drum—a typical otitis media case. The child fit the criteria for a *Calc carb* homeopathic remedy. In addition he was given mullein ear drops, 500 mg of vitamin C every three or four hours and the herb Echinacea. The student on call was also able to massage the pharyngeal outlet of the Eustachian tube. When I saw the child along with the student four days later, the mother reported that in ten hours the child had fallen asleep. Moreover, the fever returned to normal, the phlegm of the cold was almost gone and the boy had become his old, cheerful self. I looked in the ear that had been bulging four days earlier, and I was amazed that it had cleared so well. It had the appearance of an eardrum that had been treated with an antibiotic for a few days.

There was no redness nor bulging; it was a little pink and dull looking. That is, it was about 89 percent healed. Incredible.

I know that about 80 percent of ear infections do not need to be treated, and that many clear by themselves, but to get such a rapid response without any antibiotics was a near miracle for my "antibiotics-for-ear-infections" trained mind. And the wonderful thing about this method is that the child's immune system has learned a thing or two about how it can handle future viral and bacterial infections. This child may not get sick again. It reminded me about my own ear infection and subsequent mastoiditis after the measles when I was a five-year-old in the pre-antibiotic days. The ENT doctor had to curette out the pus-filled mastoid cells. It was a sad and painful week for me, but I've never been sick since (until I began to eat hospital food in my internship).

I am increasingly impressed with natural methods of dealing with bronchitis, skin infections, bladder infections and many other illnesses thought to involve bacteria. It is a valid approach that deserves our special consideration.

Nutrition plays an important role in this regard. The influence of nutrients on health is obvious to most of us who take supplements (it is also verified by research). The more the food industry purifies the farmers' goods so the products are sweet and stay on the grocers' shelves forever, the sicker we become. Even the Department of Agriculture back in 1933 admitted that the U.S. topsoil had been washed and blown away and the trace minerals—which are needed for optimum health—were just about gone. The farmers have found that if they put phosphates, nitrates, and potash on the soil, the plants will be big and beautiful, but the minerals and vitamins needed for human health rre often sorely lacking.

I believe our alkalinizing diet and our nutrient-deficient bodies contribute to the development of allergies, chronic fatigue, arthritis, and crime, as well as overreaction to pollutants, additives, perfumes, and modern living. If we eat properly, take the proper supplements, and control our acid/base balance, the enzymes are able to function and diseases will be less common. To a certain extent, we do not need to know the name of the disease, we only need to balance our body chemistry. If we give the body what it needs to function, and keep the ratios of the minerals and vitamins in the proper proportions, the body will heal itself. Couple this with exercise, a healthy attitude and a balanced lifestyle and we can be free of many of our 20th century maladies.

Whenever I am on the radio, television, or giving a lecture I hear story after story from people who relate their disturbing medical histories. Their doctors were only interested in making a diagnosis and treating with a drug, usually an antibiotic. There does not seem to be any interest in finding the reason for the sickness.

I believe sickness is an opportunity. It means the owner of the body was not careful (or perhaps was given poor advice) and some nasty virus, germ, or degenerative disease slipped in to tell the owner that he was doing something wrong. Sickness is not an antibiotic nor a tranquilizer deficiency. It is a sign that some biochemical tilt has occurred.

There are reasons for everything. This book is a big start. It needs to get out to the public, who should have more of a voice in the treatment of their own illness.

Lendon H. Smith, M.D.
Portland, Oregon
1992

Preface

Each person I know, each parent, each spouse, each relative, and, yes, each reader of this book would like to know they can *make a difference*. They want to be a good mother or father, a better citizen. They want to improve the lot of their family, community, church, workplace, school or college.

My claim to making a difference comes from my work as an educator, writer and family doctor who developed the concept of "The Activated Patient." I have been called the "George Washington of medical self care" and over 20 years have directly or indirectly trained an estimated 100,000 people with such skills. I have described in my dozen or so books these three self care assumptions:

1. Lay people supplied with clear, simple information can safely handle many uncomplicated ills, injuries and emergencies earlier, cheaper and sometimes better than health care professionals.

2. Those with little formal education can be trusted just as much as the highly educated to wisely deal with common conditions.

3. Medical and nursing knowledge need not and should not be closely guarded secrets of the health professional, but should be shared lay persons.

Such concepts and philosophies have been the uniting force behind us as Dr. Schmidt, Dr. Smith and myself came together to write *Beyond Antibiotics*. You must become Activated Patients in a very direct way. When your doctor says:

... "Here's your prescription for the antibiotic for you/your child."

or

     ... "I think this *might* be a strep throat, take this."

or

     ... "Just to be on the safe side, take this amoxicillin for ten days."

You must have more to say than, "Thanks, doctor." You must clear your throat, look the doctor straight in the eyes and learn to say:

     ... "Are you sure this is a *bacterial* infection and not a viral or fungal infection (which are not susceptible to antibiotics)?"

or

     ... "Have you ordered a culture and sensitivity from the lab to determine what kind of bacterial infection is present?"

or

     ... "I'd rather not take an antibiotic. Is there something else I can do (like the things we describe in our book)?"

For some people as they deal with the fast-paced and rapidly-changing medical world, that is tough to do. If you are a young parent, a "working mom" or someone who is looking to the doctor for a quick fix, a "silver bullet," such questions may be considered disrespectful or just plain unnecessary. Doesn't your doctor know what's best for you? Isn't that what you are paying him/her for? Maybe your pediatrician/family doctor/internist is not into this "health partnership" business. Perhaps they don't think kindly of people who come in with the latest *Reader's Digest* article on health. Perhaps your M.D. is too busy to think about cultures and extra requisitions. Besides, didn't he/she just come from that big medical meeting with an update on the latest and strongest (and perhaps *most expensive*) antibiotic? Aren't you really too busy earning a living, taking care of kids, cleaning the house to bother with extra reading and thinking?

As you think this over you might ask, "How is it that you authors know so much about antibiotics anyway?"

Well, one advantage I have is that I've been doctoring longer than most of today's doctors—for over 40 years. I've seen trends;

I've gained experience as a researcher, professor and clinician. I worked *inside* the pharmaceutical industry as medical director of a major Swiss drug firm. I was a professor at both Georgetown School of Medicine and the University of Minnesota School of Medicine. I've learned how drug studies are done, how universities make grant applications and do research. I've done many clinical studies myself.

I have also never forgotten the pledge I took when I graduated from medical school, *Primum non nocera* (first, do no harm). *Help* the patient if you can, but don't hurt them in the process. I remember the early days of antibiotic therapy (1950–1965) when we were advised to routinely use *Lactobacillus acidophilus* to compensate for antibiotic overkill. I read the warnings of Sir Alexander Fleming (the man who discovered penicillin) about the development of bacterial resistance to antibiotics. I recall the first patient I had who developed an allergic reaction to penicillin, and nearly died. I have vivid memories of the death of the wife of one of our local bankers who did die after she took the powerful antibiotic, chloromycitin.

I have had my little granddaughter given a prescription for 10 days of amoxicillin because she had a "red ear" at six months of age. When her mother confronted the pediatrician about the wisdom of such advice she was told, "If you don't like what I tell you, go get another doctor!" (Incidentally, the baby did *not* take the antibiotic and the "red ear" disappeared as soon as her first tooth came in two days later!)

Such experiences have made me leery of using antibiotics over the years. It culminated in a recent survey I made of 3,000 patients I have treated for candida-related complex (CRC). Over 90 percent of the patients reported excessive and prolonged use of broad-spectrum antibiotics prior to the onset of this common yeast-related illness—a problem that frequently produces sinusitis, ear infections, gastrointestinal dysfunction, depression, hormonal problems, mental confusion, chronic fatigue and vaginitis (in women). Most of these patients took antibiotics prescribed in good faith by their doctors, but what was meant to be *helpful* turned out to be *harmful.*

So, as you prepare to read *Beyond Antibiotics,* I ask you to become Activated Patients. Investigate what you can do to improve your nutritional and immunological resources. Become curious about options you can use instead of antibiotics. Become evangelistic as you tell others about what you've learned.

It will help *you make a difference.*

Keith W. Sehnert, M.D.
Minneapolis, MN
1992

I

Are Antibiotics the Best Medicine?

1

Casualties of
the War on Germs

"Half of what we have taught you is wrong. Unfortunately, we do
not know which half."

Dean Burwell, M.D., addressing
medical students at Harvard University[1]

You've come down with a cold, the flu, a sore throat, a cough, sinus
congestion or perhaps a bladder infection. The symptoms are
sufficiently bothersome that you choose to go to the doctor. You
already know what that doctor is likely to do—prescribe an antibiotic for ten days. For some individuals in this predicament, the
antibiotic does its work and the problem is gone. For others, the initial symptoms are unaffected and are now accompanied by unwanted side effects. For yet others, the antibiotic treatment results in
aggravation of their health, perhaps even in chronic problems. For
those still less fortunate, antibiotic is followed by antibiotic in a
seemingly endless effort to kill the alleged invaders.

Antibiotics are prescribed at an alarming rate in this country.
Obstetricians and gynecologists write 2,645,000 antibiotic prescriptions every *week*. Internists give out 1,416,000 in the same
period.[2,3] Pediatricians and family physicians lead the way, prescribing over $500 million worth of antibiotics each year to treat just
one problem—ear infections in children. Another $500 million-
plus is spent on antibiotics to treat other pediatric illness.[4] Over
the past 15 years, antibiotic prescriptions to young children have

risen a staggering 51 percent.[5] Antibiotics continue to be prescribed for conditions that do not even warrant their use.

This heavy prescribing of antibiotics is not without costs in both dollars and human suffering. Perhaps the worst tragedy is that many doctors consider much of the antibiotic prescribing medically unnecessary or worse—harmful! Consider the views expressed by leaders in the fields of infectious diseases and medical consumerism, much of which has been published in medical textbooks and peer-reviewed medical journals:

- "After Congressional hearings and numerous academic studies on this issue, it has become the general consensus that 40 to 60 percent of all antibiotics in this country are misprescribed."[6]

- "Pharyngitis and tonsillitis . . . are among the worst-treated of all illnesses, primarily because of the overprescription of antibiotics."[7]

- "In 1983, more than 51 percent of the more than 3 million patients who saw doctors for treatment of the common cold were unnecessarily given a prescription for an antibiotic."[8] Antibiotics do nothing for the common cold because the condition is viral in nature.

- "It is no accident that the most allergic generation in history has been raised on antibiotics. Several times a week I see a new patient whose allergies appeared or became much worse after a course of antibiotics."[9]

- "Researchers are questioning whether the routine use of antibiotics is a contributing factor to frequently occurring acute otitis media [middle ear infection] and persistent middle ear fluid—conditions that were rare before the advent of antimicrobial therapy."[10]

- "Recurrence rates [of middle ear fluid] were significantly higher in the antibiotic-treated group than in the placebo group." Children receiving amoxicillin for chronic middle ear infection experienced two to six times the rate of recurrence.[11]

- Antibiotics used to treat upper respiratory infections have been shown to *cause* urinary tract infections.[12]

- Antibiotics can disrupt the vaginal flora, making the patient more susceptible to vaginal infections such as that due to the yeast *Candida albicans.*[13]
- *"Candida albicans* infection, often associated with antibiotic-induced alterations in microbial flora, may cause defects in cellular immunity."[14]

While no one can argue the fact that antibiotics have saved lives, many authorities believe that doctors' efforts to "eradicate microbes at all costs" represent an undeclared war that is not without a price. In fact, some suggest there are numerous circumstances in which the risks of antibiotics outweigh the benefits.

The War on Germs

The war on germs was declared when doctors first realized that bacteria were associated with various illnesses, and antibiotics then became available that were effective in killing bacteria. This war was pursued with vigor for some 50 years and has yet to show signs of relenting. As with any war, there are casualties. However, the casualties are often the patients, not just the germs.

In pre-antibiotic days, hospital beds were largely occupied by people with pneumonia complicated with pleurisy and empyema, typhoid fever, osteomyelitis, peritonsillar abscesses, peritonitis, and furuncles, boils and other pus-filled sequelae of infections and accidents. It was smelly and messy. The discovery of penicillin and the ensuing quick cascade of antibiotic formulations propelled the medical profession out of the bed-side hand-holding empathic method into the aggressive modern therapeutic paradigm.

Doctors believed it was safe and appropriate to give antibiotics to anyone who looked like he may be coming down with an infected ear or whose post-nasal drip might turn into pneumonia. If a patient happened to be in the hospital, it was almost axiomatic that he would get an antibiotic. Hospitalized patients got secondary infections while in for "observation" of their heart attack, control of diabetes, or a viral respiratory infection, for example. Antibiotics were prescribed prophylactically (preventively) in the majority of patients. After about five years of this method of "covering" the possibilities, hospitals began to report the increased incidence of secondary infections, *despite* the routine use of these antibiotics. While there were many medical miracles and many lives saved by the prudent use of antibiotics, there came a mounting list of casualties.

Case 1: Jeff was a 13-year-old boy who complained of pain in his lower right abdomen and began to run a fever of 101 degrees. The white blood cell count was 12,000, almost twice normal, and he had tenderness and guarding in the right lower quadrant of his belly. The surgeon agreed that it must be a "hot" appendix. He operated and was chagrined to find a normal appendix. The boy was sent home in a few days after the wound healed, but something went wrong. The symptoms he experienced before the surgery had returned. The mother called Dr. Smith about a week after the surgery. "Can someone have two appendices?" she queried.

No one had heard of this anomaly—two appendices! What was going on? Everything was as it was before Jeff got sick. The only thing his mother could recall was that the boy had resumed his anti-acne antibiotic (erythromycin), which had been interrupted by the hospital stay. Dr. Smith suggested that the boy quit the antibiotic for a while and see what happens. It worked. When he was off the antibiotic he was free of symptoms. Every time he began the erythromycin, he got a bellyache.

Case 2: Mark was a 26-year-old man who had suffered as a child from recurrent tonsillitis and ear infections. For seven years of his life, he was on antibiotics almost constantly to "prevent" and treat tonsillitis. At age 12, he developed severe acne. From age 12 to age 18 he was on tetracycline. There was little improvement in his acne, yet Mark's dermatologist was convinced antibiotics were the solution. Mark began to lose weight and to suffer from diarrhea and chronic fatigue.

Mark was not a healthy adult by any means. He was at least 35 pounds underweight in spite of a ravenous appetite. He had multiple food sensitivities and physical signs of nutritional deficiency. He was tired most of the day, could not exercise without pain, and found it difficult to work a full day without sleeping for a couple of hours after lunch. He had been to countless doctors in his search for solutions, with little success.

Casualties of the War on Germs

Mark's most prominent symptom was diarrhea which had persisted for years without relenting. He had seven to eight bowel movements a day, all of which were loose. Mark was found to have a profound disruption of the normal intestinal bacteria, with an overgrowth of the yeast *Candida albicans* and an infection by the parasite *Giardia lamblia*. Mark was a casualty of the war on germs. His immune system had been disrupted, his intestinal tract damaged, and he became susceptible to all kinds of opportunistic bugs.

Case 3: Karen was a 33-year-old secretary. She had recurrent tonsillitis and ear infections as a child for which antibiotics were prescribed liberally. Her comment "I was on antibiotics more than I was off them" is a common theme in such patients. At about age 12, she developed recurrent bladder infections which were treated using sulfonamides. The bladder infections continued off and on throughout her adult life. She also suffered from recurrent vaginal yeast infections, which had been treated with antibiotics.

At age 22, Karen developed acne vulgaris, which is a serious form of acne where large pustules riddle the face. Her physicians treated her acne with tetracycline. Whenever she received a dose of antibiotic, her vaginitis became severe. She reacted adversely to most foods eaten. Remarkably, her body swelled like a balloon, gaining 10 pounds of fluid within days.

Karen also suffered from severe depression which was aggravated markedly while she was on antibiotics. When she felt an infection coming on, she dreaded the trip to her doctor for yet another prescription because she knew that within one or two days, she would plunge into deep depression. She was caught in a vicious cycle. Because of repeated infections of the ears, tonsils, bladder and vagina, her doctors prescribed antibiotics. The antibiotics had a short-term effect upon her symptoms, but caused her health to plummet downward.

Case 4: Brooks developed his first earache at nine months of age. He received antibiotics, which appeared to clear up the problem. In three weeks the earache returned. Antibiotics again seemed to solve the problem. This cycle of earaches and antibiotics continued for 16 months. Meanwhile, Brooks began to develop allergies to foods. After eating beans he would vomit. He had severe diarrhea from bread and headaches from fruit. As time passed he became sensitive to pollen, dust and mold, all of which aggravated his ear problems, which required more antibiotics. Brooks was on a vicious merry-go-round from which he could not exit.

Brooks' behavior began to change. He was put on Ritalin for his emergent hyperactive behavior, but this seemed to further aggravate his allergies. At age seven, Brooks once entered a room and within moments began to throw a tantrum, storming into the hallway with his hands covering his nose. When his mother asked what the problem was he shouted, "It's that varnish in the room. It gives me a bad headache!" Sure enough, the trim in the room had been varnished some two months previously. No one but the highly chemically sensitive Brooks could detect it. All of his problems seemed to begin with the multiple rounds of antibiotics. He developed intestinal problems that led to allergies. The allergies led to nutritional problems that influenced his behavior and immunity. His immune system became overwhelmed by the things in his environment to which he was exposed.

The fundamental lesson in these cases is that antibiotics were not a solution. Not only did the antibiotics fail to correct the patients' problems and actually aggravated their health, but the underlying reasons for their illness went untreated.

The war on germs has also led to more serious immediate consequences. An article in the British medical journal, *The Lancet,* reported on an outbreak of serious penicillin-resistant infections of *Haemophilus influenzae* among hospitalized children in Dallas, Texas.[15,16] *Haemophilus influenzae* is a bacterium responsible for some cases of ear infections, meningitis and epiglottitis. It was discovered that those contracting the infection were *twice* as likely to have been treated with antibiotics in the month preceding admission than were hospitalized children who did not get the infection.

The war on germs in the animal population has potentially serious consequences for humans as well. Antibiotics are used as growth enhancers and to prevent the spread of disease among chickens, turkeys, pigs and cattle. In 1983, a Midwestern outbreak of intestinal disease in 18 people was associated with an antibiotic-resistant form of *Salmonella newport* (resistant to ampicillin, carbenicillin and tetracycline). The source of the infection was traced to hamburger in which chlortetracycline had been used for growth promotion. (The use of this antibiotic led to the development of antibiotic-resistant *S. newport*.) Twelve of the people had been taking penicillin-derived antibiotics in the 24- to 48-hour period before the onset of intestinal symptoms.

According to scientists at the State Health Department in Minnesota and North Dakota, the patients had been infected before they took antibiotics. Their use of antibiotics, to which the *S. newport* was resistant, led to a reduction in the normal intestinal bacteria, resulting in more serious intestinal infection.

Researchers in charge of this case concluded that ". . . antimicrobial-resistant organisms of animal origin cause serious human illness," and urged ". . . far more prudent use of antimicrobials in both humans and animals."[17]

Ask the Right Questions

It is odd that billions of dollars are spent on the development of new antibiotics to kill bacteria associated with infections, but no one seems to be interested in asking the vital question, "What is it that renders us susceptible or resistant to infection?" Why does Ed frequently succumb to bronchitis, sinus infections and colds while his wife Emily never gets sick? Why does Megan get repeated vaginal and respiratory infections, while her sister Amy, who stays out late and eats poorly, remains untouched by such illness?

Most researchers today are asking "How can we kill this bacteria" or "How can we prevent the spread of that bacteria," and this is fine. There is value in asking and answering these questions. But far too many doctors and researchers almost completely ignore the more important issue of factors that influence susceptibility. A classic example is tonsillitis. Doctors have called this one of the worst-treated of all illnesses because of the overprescription of antibiotics. Indeed, up to 80 percent of all cases of tonsillitis are due to viruses against which antibiotics have no impact. It is common for people to have the strep bacteria in their throat yet have no evidence of illness whatsoever. These people have been dubbed "carriers" because they carry the germ but don't become ill. They are thought to be able to pass the infection on to other people, but they themselves are unaffected. Why do they remain well despite the presence of large numbers of "disease-causing" organisms in their bodies? What is peculiar to their immune systems that renders them unaffected? What is unusual about their diet and lifestyle that keeps them free of illness? If bacteria "cause" disease, these people should become sick, yet they don't. During epidemics of tonsillitis, the number of carriers in the population may reach an astonishing 60 percent. *Yet we spend virtually no time studying these people.*[18]

Perhaps it is because our medical system is intent on studying *disease* rather than health. It is interested in spending money and resources on learning about pathology rather than wellness. (As one medical analyst said, "There is more money to be made in searching for a cure than in finding one.") This view is exemplified in an encounter described by Russell Jaffe, M.D., Ph.D., former researcher with the National Institutes of Health (NIH) and a current leader in the field of preventive medicine. Some years ago, Dr. Jaffe approached the director of NIH noting that some 125 divisions of NIH are devoted to the study of disease, but *not one* was dedicated to the study of health. Dr. Jaffe proposed that a new division be opened at NIH specifically for the purpose of studying health, which is a very different endeavor than studying disease. This division, Jaffe suggested, would investigate the biology, physiology, biochemistry and psychology of people who remain healthy to learn what makes them unique. Knowledge of such people could then be applied to people with illness in order to prevent disease. Jaffe was cordially told that the National Institutes of Health was doing just fine studying disease and that there was no reason to study health. Since then, Dr. Jaffe has said rather tongue-in-cheek that perhaps they should change the name to the National Institutes of *Disease.*[19]

With the discovery of new germs each year, the effort to find a specific drug to kill them all grows more futile. More and more research is revealing that diet, nutrition, environment, lifestyle, habits, attitude and stress have a profound effect on our immunity and resistance to disease. The National Cancer Institute has proclaimed that 60 to 70 percent of all cancer, which is deeply rooted in the immune system, is related to diet, lifestyle and environment. Physician and researcher Thomas McKeown summarizes nicely the broader view of infectious illness and the arrogance involved in suspecting that man can combat it with a pill. He states, ". . . the conclusion which seems inescapable is that the influences which determine man's response to infectious disease—genetics, nutritional, environmental, behavioral, as well as medical—are infinitely complex, and we need to be very cautious before assuming that we fully understand the infection, or that we have in our hands the certain means of their control."[20]

This book is about boosting immunity and improving resistance to infections and disease in general. We ask "the right questions" and provide helpful answers in areas of life known to affect immunity. But before looking into this mystery, it is important to understand why antibiotics are problematic and why their use should be reduced.

2

Antibiotics:
What Your Doctor
May Not Tell You

"Deaths from common infections were declining long before effective medical intervention was possible."
Thomas McKeown, M.D.
The Role of Medicine[1]

Around the turn of this century, cholera claimed the lives of hundreds of thousands of people. Medicine seemed almost helpless in the face of this epidemic. Most doctors blamed the cholera bacterium for these ravages on the population, but all were not convinced. Many doctors believed that a healthy person would not become sick and die merely because of exposure to the bacteria. They believed more was required. Some endeavored to prove it.

As Bernard Dixon reports in *Beyond the Magic Bullet*, "Around 1900, when he was 74, a Bavarian doctor, Max von Pettenkofer, knowingly consumed a culture containing millions of cholera bacilli, isolated from a fatal case of the disease. At about the same time the Russian pathologist Elie Metchnikoff conducted the same bizarre experiment. So did several of their colleagues. Some of the intrepid experimenters experienced mild diarrhea. All had enormous numbers of cholera bacilli in their faeces. But none developed anything like cholera. Metchnikoff is celebrated as the discoverer of . . . white blood cells which can engulf and destroy invading germs. His life's work centered upon the healing power of the body in its battles against infection. Metchnikoff . . . taught that the correct way to deal with infectious disease was not by administering chemicals but by strengthening and, where necessary, exploiting the body's own defenses."[2]

This view was in stark contrast to that of Louis Pasteur, who believed a germ could be found for every malady. He contended that if the germ could be isolated and a treatment devised to kill the germ, virtually all disease might someday be eradicated. Indeed, history has remembered Pasteur as the father of microbiology. Yet, in the final years of his life, Pasteur came to realize that his theories about germs were erroneous. Just prior to his death, he is said to have uttered the words "The terrain is everything, the bacteria is nothing."[3] Pasteur recognized that it was not bacteria that were responsible for disease, but the "terrain" (the surrounding land), the inability of the host to combat them. If the host was "strong" (i.e., the immune system was active), the organisms could not get a foothold. If the host was weak, the organisms could "settle in" and "overcome." Pasteur had come to the conclusion that myriad factors, including diet, nutrition, stress, heredity, environment and state of mind, had a profound effect on resistance to microbes.

The view of infectious disease was divided into two camps: those who adhered to Pasteur's original germ theory and those who believed health of the host was more important. The discovery of sulfa drugs and penicillin in the 1930s and 1940s launched medicine fully into the chemotherapeutic approach to infection and all but laid to waste the notion of host resistance. Thus was born the Antibiotic Age.

The Paradoxes of Antibiotic Use

The American Heritage Dictionary of the English Language defines paradox as "a situation or action exhibiting inexplicable or contradictory aspects." There are inherent contradictory aspects associated with the use of antibiotics. They are used to aid the body in fighting infection but may actually give rise to or encourage the development of recurrent infections, thus increasing the reliance upon antibiotics. They kill bacteria, but can foster the development of bacteria resistant to antibiotics. Because of this, diseases once responsive to antibiotics can no longer be treated with those same antibiotics. In addition, antibiotics are used to bridge the gap in times of insufficient immune response, yet they may undermine the immune response. Moreover, antibiotics are frequently not appropriate, yet doctors are discouraged from using alternatives.

The greatest paradox of all may be that persistence in using antibiotics and pursuit of newer and newer antibiotic drugs have drawn attention away from other means of managing infections. This pursuit has consumed valuable research dollars that might have been used to develop methods that stimulate immune function, or to discover why some of us get sick while others remain well.

Antibiotics and Infection: Not What You Think

Antibiotics are rightly credited with saving countless lives over the past 40 years that might have been lost to overwhelming infection. Sulfanilamide was effective against specific forms of bacterial infections such as pneumococcal pneumonia. This was followed by the introduction of penicillin, which proved to be nearly miraculous in its effect upon stubborn bacterial diseases. Today, antibiotics save lives, reduce suffering and will continue to do so. Yet, these "miracle drugs" can hardly be given credit for the general decline of infectious diseases. The incidence of tuberculosis, rheumatic fever, pneumonia, diphtheria, scarlet fever, whooping cough and typhoid had declined substantially before the introduction of antibiotics. Antibiotics did not appear to cause further decline in these diseases. According to epidemiologist R. R. Porter, "Nearly 90 percent of the total decline in the death rate during this epoch [1860–1965] had occurred prior to the introduction of antibiotics."[4]

According to Dr. Thomas McKeown, physician and professor of social hygiene at the University of Birmingham in England ". . . the decline in mortality in the second half of the 19th century was due wholly to a reduction of deaths from infectious diseases; there was no evidence of a decline in other causes of death. Examination of the diseases which contributed to the decline suggested that the main influences were: (a) rising standards of living, of which the most significant feature was a better diet; (b) improvements in hygiene; and (c) a favorable trend in the relationship between some micro-organisms and the human host. *Therapy* [medical treatment] *made no contributions,* and the effect of immunization was restricted to smallpox, which accounted for only about one twentieth of the reduction of the death rate." [emphasis added][5] McKeown cites tuberculosis as one example. He writes, "By the time streptomycin was introduced, mortality from the disease had fallen to a small fraction of its level during 1848 to 1854. . . . Its contribution to the decrease in the death rate since the early 19th century was only about 3 percent."[6]

In a presidential address to the Infectious Diseases Society of America in 1971, infectious disease expert Dr. E. H. Kass argued that most of the decline in mortality for most infectious conditions occurred prior to the discovery of either "the cause" of the disease or some purported "treatment" for it.[7] Dr. Kass appears to be saying that finding bacteria associated with a disease and the ensuing antibiotic treatment had little or no impact on the decline of infectious diseases. This is in agreement with other researchers.

John B. McKinlay and Sonja M. McKinlay, researchers at Boston University, have done an extensive analysis of the impact of medical treatment on infectious disease. Regarding ten common infectious diseases, their analysis suggests that ". . . at most, 3.5 percent of the total decline in mortality since 1900 could be ascribed to medical measures introduced for the diseases considered here." They conclude, "In general, medical measures (both chemotherapeutic and prophylactic) appear to have contributed little to the overall decline in mortality in the United States since about 1900— having in many instances been introduced several decades after a marked decline had already set in and having no detectable influence in most instances."[8] Marc Lappé, Ph.D., professor at the University of Illinois, suggests similarly that "no antibiotic can be said to have proven successful in truly eradicating any infectious disease in modern times."[11]

Writing in the *Journal of Infectious Disease,* Dr. L. Weinstein points out that despite the supposed value of antibiotics, the incidence and mortality of many infectious conditions (such as subacute

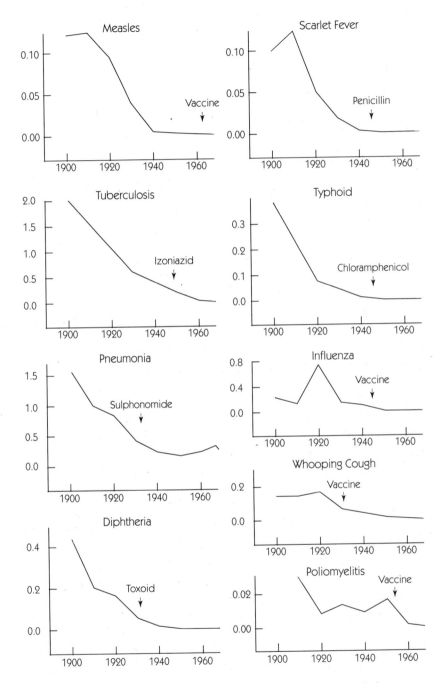

The Fall in the Standardized Death Rate (per 1,000 population) for Nine Common Infectious Diseases in Relation to Specific Medical Measures, for the United States, 1900–1973. Reprinted with permission, *Millbank Memorial Fund Quarterly,* 1977.[9,10]

bacterial endocarditis, streptococcal pharyngitis, pneumococcal pneumonia, gonorrhea and syphilis) have actually increased. He notes, somewhat paradoxically, that the incidence and mortality of other diseases such as chickenpox have decreased in the absence of any treatment.[12]

So what are we to make of this evidence? While antibiotics have undeniably proven valuable on a case-by-case basis, there are serious questions regarding whether they are responsible for past declines in infectious disease or whether they will be the means by which current or future declines in infectious disease are realized. Having raised these questions about the value and effectiveness of antibiotics, at least from a historical perspective, we must take a close look at a variety of problems presented today by the use of antibiotics.

The Perils of Antibiotic Use

For decades we have heard of the miracles brought about by antibiotic treatment. Lately, doctors have begun to more seriously explore the problems associated with antibiotic use. In this section we look at many of the problems that can result from antibiotic use and overuse. This presentation may seem biased because we give little consideration to the benefits of antibiotics. But the purpose of this book is to point out the fallacies and weaknesses of antibiotic drugs as they are used today. We do not deny the benefits of antibiotics and would be among the first to admit their inherent value. Our effort is to bring about changes in the way antibiotics are used and changes in the overall approach to infections.

Antibiotic-Resistant Bacteria

Antibiotics work by interfering in some way with the life cycle or metabolism of bacteria. Some antibiotics interfere with the manufacture of the cell wall. Others mimic certain natural substances that confuse the bacteria. Others disrupt the bacteria's biochemical machinery. Unfortunately, bacteria are very crafty characters. It takes them little time to adapt to our most sophisticated attempts at thwarting their advances. They do so by changing their chemistry and genes in such a way that the antibiotic has little or no effect.

Since they multiply so rapidly, they can evolve many generations in just hours. These new generations are resistant to our drugs so we must develop newer, more sophisticated antibiotics to keep up. This pursuit has perpetuated a cycle of having to constantly develop new drugs to remain one step ahead of the bacterial world.

The man who discovered penicillin, Alexander Fleming, warned that overuse of this new miracle drug might lead to problems with resistant bacteria. But his words seem to have been given little heed. According to Harvard professor and Nobel Laureate Walter Gilbert, "There may be a time down the road when 80 percent to 90 percent of infections will be resistant to all known antibiotics."[13] A chilling thought.

Unfortunately, Dr. Gilbert's warnings may be giving way to reality. According to Dr. Richard Krause, senior scientific advisor to the National Institutes of Health and former director of the National Institute of Allergies and Infectious Diseases, "We have an epidemic of microbial resistance." An article in *Science* (August 1992), one of the world's leading scientific journals, provides this somber assessment: ". . . doctors in hospitals and clinics around the world are losing the battle against an onslaught of new drug-resistant bacterial infections including staph, pneumonia, strep, tuberculosis, dysentery, and other diseases that are costly and difficult, if not impossible, to treat."*

Dr. Schmidt reported in his book *Childhood Ear Infections* that "the trend in bacterial development of antibiotic resistance is not unlike the increasing resistance of agricultural pests to pesticides. In 1938, scientists knew of just *seven* insect and mite species that had acquired resistance to pesticides. By 1984 that figure had climbed to 447 and included most of the world's major pests. In response to heavier pesticide use and a wider variety of pesticides, pests have evolved sophisticated mechanisms for resisting the action of chemicals designed to kill them. Pesticides also kill the pests' natural enemies, much like antibiotics kill the natural enemies of harmful bacteria in the body."[14]

The trouble with antibiotics is that the weaker, more susceptible

---

*Exploring new strategies to fight drug-resistant microbes. *Science* 1992; 257:1036-1038.

bacteria are usually killed while the *hearty* bacteria develop resistance. In the words of Gilbert H. Welch, M.D., a specialist in the study of antibiotic resistance, ". . . antibiotic use, while contributing to the immediate demise of bacteria, serves to 'educate' microbes by establishing selective pressure that favors the 'smarter' bacteria, i.e., those that can resist the antibiotic."[15] Darwin would call this "survival of the fittest."

If Dr. Welch's contention is true, we would expect those who have received repeated doses of a particular antibiotic to harbor more bacteria that are resistant to that antibiotic. This is indeed the case. In *Drug Information,* published by the American Hospital Formulary Service, it states that "children who have received repeated doses of ampicillin, or other antibiotics in the penicillin group, harbor more antibiotic-resistant *Haemophilus influenzae* than those with little or no exposure to these drugs."[16] *(Haemophilus influenzae* is a bacterium associated with ear infections and meningitis.)

When children harbor antibiotic-resistant bacteria as a result of prior antibiotic therapy, the consequences can sometimes be severe. An article in the British medical journal, *Lancet,* reported on an outbreak of serious penicillin-resistant infections of *H. influenzae* among hospitalized children in Dallas, Texas. It was discovered that those contracting the infection were *twice* as likely to have been treated with antibiotics in the month preceding admission than were hospitalized children who did not get the infection.[17] From 1975 to 1977 the number of antibiotic-resistant strains of *H. influenzae* rose by almost 35 percent.[18] The medical literature has other similar accounts.

The bane of antibiotic resistance has affected nearly every form of bacteria known to cause disease in humans. It has even caused previously harmless bacteria to become disease-producing. The common intestinal bacteria *E. coli* has long been a normal inhabitant of the human intestinal tract. But, as a result of the widespread use of antibiotics, some *E. coli* have mutated into a more virulent form that has been implicated in bladder infections, diarrhea and a variety of other human ills.

Gonorrhea was once quickly and easily treated with penicillin. However, as more strains developed resistance to penicillin, larger and larger doses were required to treat the disease. Other antibiotics such as tetracycline were also used. Today these drugs, formerly the cornerstones of treatment, are only minimally effective in treating gonorrhea. In September 1990, officials from the Centers for Disease Control issued a statement that penicillin and tetracycline *should be abandoned as a treatment for gonorrhea* because of a sharp rise in the numbers of bacteria resistant to these drugs.[19] The CDC now recommend the use of the more toxic and more costly cefoxitin and spectinomycin.

Harold C. Neu, professor of medicine and pharmacology at Columbia University, wrote a paper in Science (August 1992) entitled "The Crisis in Antibiotic Resistance." In this article, he points out that in 1941, only 40,000 units of penicillin per day for four days were required to *cure* pneumococcal pneumonia. "Today," says Neu, "a patient could receive 24 million units of penicillin a day and die of pneumococcal meningitis." He adds that bacteria that cause infection of the respiratory tract, skin, bladder, bowel and blood ". . . are now resistant to virtually all of the older antibiotics. The extensive use of antibiotics in the community and hospitals has fueled this crises."*

Mitchell L. Cohen, a researcher with the National Center for Infectious Diseases at the Centers for Disease Control, issued this warning about antibiotics in 1992: "Unless currently effective antimicrobial agents can be successfully preserved and the transmission of drug-resistant organisms curtailed, the post-antimicrobial era may be rapidly approaching in which infectious disease wards housing untreatable conditions will again be seen."† Patients, doctors, scientists and public health officials must all play their part in finding ways to reduce reliance upon antibiotics.

Destruction of Friendly Bacteria

We have been conditioned to perceive all bacteria as "bad." Indeed, bacteria such as *Haemophilus influenzae* and *Streptococcus pneumoniae,* encountered in common upper respiratory infections, are

---

*Neu, HC. The crisis in antibiotic resistance. *Science* 1992;257:1064-1073.
†Cohen, ML. Epidemiology of drug resistance: implications for a post-antimicrobial era. *Science* 1992;257:1050-1055.

for the most part "bad guys." However, we would probably die from all sorts of opportunistic infections if not for the "good" bacteria. These bacteria live in the mouth, on the skin, in the vagina and in the intestinal tract. Bacteria that normally live on your skin, for example, secrete substances that protect against bacterial and fungal infections of the skin. *Lactobacillus* bacteria living in the gut and the vagina help protect against invasion by yeast and other germs.

The intestinal tract is home to countless different varieties of microbes, most of which live in harmony together. They exist in what scientists call a *symbiotic* relationship, meaning they benefit from the existence of one another. Most people are surprised to learn that microbes in the intestinal tract outnumber the *total* number of cells in the human body by a factor of 10! The functions performed by many of these organisms are vital to optimum health.

The bacterium *Lactobacillus acidophilus* is one of the more important beneficial bacteria. It plays a role in the digestion of food and the manufacture of vitamins B_1, B_2, B_3, B_{12} and folic acid. It also secretes substances that destroy invading infectious bacteria, parasites and fungi (e.g. acidophilin, a natural antibiotic, various organic acids and peroxides). *Bifidobacterium bifidus* is another important intestinal bacterium, especially in children. One reason breastfed children suffer from fewer intestinal infections than bottlefed children is the high number of *Bifidobacteria* in the intestines of breastfed babies. When breastfeeding is discontinued, the number of *Bifidobacteria* (Bifidus) in the intestine decreases dramatically.

Another way that the normal intestinal bacteria protect against infection by invaders is by occupying space. They attach themselves to the wall of the intestines, leaving no available space to which parasites and other organisms can attach. If the good bacteria are eliminated, opportunists can move in and set up shop. The opportunists compete with the other intestinal organisms for nutrients. Worse, they rob nutrients from the host. As they gain a stronger hold, they make it easier for other members of their species to invade and get a foothold—they multiply. This reduces the integrity of the intestinal tract, sometimes called a "leaky gut," increases the chance of developing allergies, and lowers the level of health. Finally, the immune response of the host is reduced.

A Minnesota biologist once said that if you had two mice, gave them all the food they needed and took away all their predators, at the end of one year there would be *one million* mice. A staggering figure, but not an unusual outcome when one disturbs the balance of Mother Nature. In a similar way, antibiotics can disrupt the balance in the intestines, leading to the overgrowth of a host of unwanted pests such as yeast.

Antibiotics and the Yeast Connection

Doctors have known for many years that antibiotics can cause yeast overgrowth. A pregnant mother is given antibiotics for her bladder infection and develops a vaginal yeast infection. She then delivers her child, who develops oral thrush—that fluffy white coating of the tongue due to yeast. According to William G. Crook, M.D., author of *The Yeast Connection,* "Broad-spectrum antibiotics resemble machine gun-shooting terrorists in a crowded airport. While they're killing enemies, they also kill friendly and innocent bystanders. In a similar manner, antibiotics knock out friendly bacteria on the interior membranes of a person's body while they're eradicating enemies. When this happens, yeasts flourish and put out a toxin that affects various organs and systems in the body, including the immune system."[20] Recently doctors at the University of Southern California found that excessive antibiotics used to treat ear infections in children contributed to the growth of yeast in the middle ear. It was only after treatment with an antifungal drug, ketoconazole, that the middle ears of these children improved.[21]

Immune suppression by way of yeast infection is another adverse effect brought about by antibiotics. In the May/June issue of *Infections in Medicine,* published in 1985, Steven S. Witkin, M.D., writes "*Candida albicans* infection, often associated with antibiotic-induced alterations in microbial flora, may cause defects in cellular immunity. . . . Recent studies suggest that the infection itself may cause immunosuppression, resulting in recurrences in certain patients. In addition to creating an increased susceptibility to the candida reinfection, the immunological alterations may also be related to subsequent endocrinopathies and autoantibody formation."[22]

Leo Galland, M.D. was the keynote speaker at a 1988 conference on candida related complex. In his address, he noted that antibiotics were a precipitating factor in 82 percent of the patients with CRC.[23]

Major symptoms of candida-related complex (CRC) include:

Fatigue or lethargy ✓	Constipation
Poor memory	Bloating, intestinal gas ✓
Feeling "spacy" or "unreal" ✓	Vaginal itching, burning, discharge ✓
Numbness, burning, tingling	Prostatitis
Insomnia	Premenstrual tension, PMS ✓
Muscle aches, weakness ✓	Attacks of anxiety or crying ✓
Abdominal pain	Shaking or irritability when hungry

Other symptoms include:

Headaches, sinusitis ✓	Food sensitivity or intolerance ✓
Moodiness ✓	Mucus in stools
White tongue	Rectal itching ✓
Tendency to bruise easily	Hoarseness, loss of voice
Chronic rashes, itching	Nasal itching ✓

Antibiotics and Chronic Fatigue Syndrome

The media has recently begun to publicize a condition known as chronic fatigue syndrome, or CFS. People with CFS suffer from myriad symptoms, which their doctors are often unable to treat. The major symptom is chronic fatigue. Such people are often unable function in a normal way. They are commonly exhausted, irritable, depressed, confused, suffer from muscle and joint pains and are unable to sleep.

In 1989 and 1990, Carol Jessop, M.D., a California researcher of CFS and Assistant Clinical Professor at the University of California at San Francisco, presented case studies of patients with chronic fatigue syndrome. She reported that 80 percent of these patients had a history of *recurrent antibiotic treatment* (as a child, adolescent or adult). William G. Crook, M.D., author of *Chronic Fatigue Syndrome and the Yeast Connection* concludes similarly that the overuse of antibiotics is a major contributing factor to the development of chronic fatigue.[24]

In 1991, David S. Bauman, Ph.D. and Howard E. Hagglund, M.D. reported in the *Journal of Advancement in Medicine,* on a study of 43 women who were classified as "Polysystem Chronic Complainers." These women suffered from 10 or more symptoms, including poor memory, fatigue, mood swings, head pressure, muscle aches, digestive symptoms and inability to concentrate. Of these 43 women, 29 (or 67%) reported having been on prolonged courses of antibiotics. Only 5 of 33 controls (reporting fewer than 4 complaints) had a history of prolonged antibiotic use.[25]

Antibiotics and Immune Suppression

One irony of antibiotic use is that while they are intended to "bolster" the immune response by killing bacteria, they may in some cases have a suppressive effect on immunity. Evidence for this comes from two basic sources: studies of the effect of antibiotics on the activity of white blood cells, and the outcome of infections treated with antibiotics.

In an article published in *The American Journal of Medicine* in 1982, Drs. William Hauser and Jack Remington of Stanford University School of Medicine reported on the ability of some antibiotics to alter the immune response. Tetracycline was shown to inhibit the ability of white cells to engulf and destroy bacteria (phagocytosis) and to delay the ability of white cells to move to the site of infection. Sulfonamides inhibited the microbiocidal activity of white cells. Trimethoprim-sulfamethoxazole inhibited antibody production. Similar action of numerous antibiotics was reported.[26]

Antibiotics have also been shown to increase the likelihood of repeat infections. In one report, children with strep throat who were given antibiotics recovered from the initial infection in short order. However, they experienced a rate of recurrent infections two to eight times higher than those not receiving antibiotics. This was especially true if antibiotics were given in the first two days of illness.[27]

Similar findings have been reported with antibiotics used to treat ear infections. A study published in 1974 showed that children with acute earaches who received antibiotics within the first few days of the illness experienced up to 2.9 times more recurrent infections than those in whom antibiotic use was delayed (7 or more days) or avoided.[28] This study was met with some skepticism and seemed to have little impact on medical practice. A 1991 article published in the *Journal of the American Medical Association* has renewed the debate raised by the 1974 study. It showed that children with chronic earaches who received antibiotics experienced two to six times more recurrent middle ear effusion than those receiving placebo.[29]

Such evidence seems to suggest that antibiotics may in some cases limit the *body's* ability to recognize and destroy invading bacteria. It appears that when antibiotic treatment is delayed, children are able to develop natural immunity, thereby insulating them from future episodes. Early antibiotic therapy may inhibit the initial immune response, which may increase the likelihood of repeat infections.

Predisposition to Infection by Parasites

For most of this century, intestinal parasites were considered (by Western standards) a disease of the Third World. Parasitic infection usually occurred in countries where hygiene was poor, water impure and human waste treatment nonexistent. Today, parasitic infection is becoming more common in the U.S. In several recent studies, from 30 to 50 percent of various childhood populations was found to harbor some kind of parasite. Parasite infection has become more common in North America for several reasons:

1) antibiotics, 2) day care, 3) foreign travel, 4) immigration, 5) water contamination of rivers, streams and public water supplies, 6) changes in fiber consumption, 7) bottlefeeding of infants and 8) overall changes in diet.

Parasites can cause fever, intestinal pain, poor absorption of nutrients and many other symptoms. These symptoms are commonly misdiagnosed as a bacterial infection and treated with antibiotics, which only serve to tighten the parasite's grip on its host.

The use of antibiotics often results in increased susceptibility to intestinal infection by fungi, bacteria, viruses and parasites because antibiotics drastically alter the balance of intestinal organisms. They kill not only the "bad guys" but also the "good guys," the friendly, helpful bacteria in the digestive tract. Two such bacterial species are _Lactobacillus acidophilus_ and _Bifidobacterium bifidus._ When these organisms are wiped out, an environment is created in the intestines that favors the growth of undesirables such as the common fungus _Candida albicans._

Marc Lappé, Ph.D., author of _When Antibiotics Fail,_ summarizes some of the intestinal effects of antibiotics as follows: "Lincomycin eliminates virtually all of the bacteria that require oxygen, while neomycin and kanamycin decrease the number of oxygen-requiring germs and gram-positive anaerobic ones, leading to overgrowth of _Candida albicans_ and _Staphylococcus aureus._ Polymyxin can reduce the native _E. Coli_ to the point of extinction, leaving the terrain open for staph and strep organisms. Erythromycin has a similar favorable effect on streptococci, while bacitracin and novobiocin lower both strep and clostridia. Ampicillin and clindamycin, by contrast, appear to favor the growth of _Clostridium dificile._"[30]

Nutrient Loss

Antibiotics can contribute to loss of important nutrients. Ironically, the nutrients that are lost because of antibiotic use are some of the same nutrients needed by the immune system to fight infection. In some cases, these same nutrients are deficient before the person becomes ill and may be one reason an infection persists.

Leo Galland, M.D., author of _Superimmunity for Kids_ and many scientific papers on nutrition and immune function, states that "Some [antibiotics] behave like magnesium sieves."[31] Antibiotics are notorious for causing diarrhea. With this diarrhea comes an important loss of nutrients. In a study of children with recurrent infections, those who experienced diarrhea had lowered magnesium levels in their blood. In these children the duration of illness was longer. According to an article published in the _Journal of Environmental Health,_ "When diarrhea lasts for a week or more, nutrient losses, anorexia, and post-enteritis malabsorption may lead to marginal malnutrition and subtle but detectable loss of immune function."[32] For example, in one kg of diarrhea—about 2 pounds, or one day's output from the "runs"—over 17 milligrams of zinc can be lost. Zinc is important in fighting both bacterial and viral infection and plays an important role in regulating inflammation. One study of people with recurrent infections showed zinc deficiency to be a problem.

Nutrient losses due to antibiotic prescribing that lasts only a week or a little more are not likely to pose any real danger. However, many children and adults are placed on antibiotics for months or years. Negative effects of this sort of treatment are more likely. As we mentioned in Chapter 1, it is not unusual for a person to report "I'm on antibiotics more than I'm off them." We've seen 5- and 6-year-old children who have spent virtually their entire lives on antibiotics. This is a tragedy!

The Food Allergy Problem

Antibiotics have also been associated with the development of food allergy or food intolerance. For many of the reasons described in previous sections, antibiotics disrupt the normal ecology and functioning of the gut. Absorption of nutrients is effected along with normal repair of the lining of the gut. Many patients of all ages have developed food allergies following antibiotic therapy. Food allergies are discussed in greater depth in Chapter 4.

Allergic Reactions

Allergic reactions are another problem associated with antibiotic use. A woman was recently admitted to Mercy Hospital in Coon Rapids, Minnesota with hives and swelling of the throat. Her airway had begun to close and would have suffocated her if not for the emergency team. She had just taken a dose of the antibiotic Keflex®. These reactions are not unexpected when you consider that in addition to the drug itself, antibiotic preparations contain sweeteners, dyes and coloring agents, flavorings and numerous unnamed excipients. In one survey of common antibiotic preparations, 85 percent contained sucrose while 34 percent contained the sweetener saccharin. Red dye #40, a coal tar derivative, was present in 45 percent of the antibiotic preparations. Many also contained FD & C yellow #5 and #6. Both of these dyes have been shown to be cross-reactive with aspirin and acetaminophen, drugs commonly taken to relieve pain and fever during infection. Moreover, FD & C yellow #5 is known to cause excessive elimination of zinc from the body.[33]

The myriad chemicals found in antibiotic preparations may or may not pose a problem for the average person. However, for those with allergies or environmental sensitivity illness (ESI), they pose a special dilemma since exposure to only tiny amounts of these synthetic substances can provoke serious reactions. For instance, yellow #5 and #6 have been associated with hives, anaphylactic shock, retching, belching, vomiting, angioneurotic edema and abdominal pain.[34] If you have allergies or are environmentally sensitive and must be on antibiotics, get a full disclosure of the contents of the particular antibiotic being considered before you use it to make sure it contains no substances to which you might react.

The Economic Cost

Antibiotics were once considered an economical means of treating infections. The benefit, treating an illness, usually outweighed the expense. As newer and more expensive antibiotics came into use for more common, less life-threatening disorders, one could argue that the cost is not always justified. There are wide disparities in the cost of antibiotics available to the consumer. For example, Keflex®, which is a brand name for the antibiotic cephalexin, costs $97 for a 10-day course of 500 mg tablets. The generic brand of the same antibiotic can be purchased for as little as $30. It seems reasonable that, given the choice between treating an infection with a $30 drug and a $97 drug of equal effectiveness, one would choose the cheaper.

There are also costs to society. For example, over $500 million are spent each year on antibiotics to treat ear infections. Studies have shown that many children receiving antibiotics for earaches have no bacteria present, meaning that antibiotics might be unnecessary in 30 to 50 percent or more of these children.[35] American doctors usually prescribe antibiotics for ten days, but recent studies of earaches have shown that two-, four-, five- and seven-day courses are equally effective.[36,37,38,39,40,41] Cutting the duration of therapy in half—as many physicians have in Holland—might reduce our tab for antibiotics considerably.

In 1983, roughly 50 percent of those receiving treatment for the common cold were given an antibiotic prescription. Yet, antibiotics do nothing for the common cold because of its viral origin.

Up to 80 percent of cases of tonsillitis are viral, yet the majority of patients receive antibiotics. This represents yet another unnecessary antibiotic expenditure. Another disorder, vaginitis, is often a direct result of antibiotic use. Many hundreds of thousands of doctor visits each year are needed to treat this disorder.

Roughly 40 percent of all antibiotics produced are used in animal husbandry. In most cases, antibiotics are used in animals raised for slaughter and eventual sale to consumers. These foods are often contaminated with antibiotic-resistant strains of *Salmonella, Campylobacter* and other strange bugs that create intestinal illness in unsuspecting diners.

Taken together, antibiotics, despite their inherent value, represent an enormous cost in personal and public health, and cost to society. As our health care costs skyrocket, doctors should carefully review the role that antibiotics might play. As is usually the case, however, consumers will probably have to be the driving force behind such change.

Bugs, Drugs and Susceptibility

The Physician's Desk Reference is used by almost all doctors to get their drug information. In the case of many of the most common antibiotics, the following recommendation is usually given: "Culture and susceptibility tests should be initiated *prior to* and *during* therapy."[42] Thus, drug manufacturers urge that doctors do a culture to determine the type of bacterium present and then test the chosen antibiotic against the bacterium—all before prescribing the antibiotic to the patient.

Unfortunately, culture and susceptibility tests are rarely done with the most common illnesses for which antibiotics are prescribed. Doctors argue that culture and susceptibility tests are impractical because their patient is ill, needs help now, and cannot wait the two or three days needed to obtain test results. Moreover, they argue, doctors usually "know" which bacteria are present. Based on this assumption, they prescribe the antibiotic.

Let's examine the problems with this logic by taking a look at ear infections, a condition which accounts for roughly 42 percent of all antibiotics prescribed to children.[43] A doctor faced with a child complaining of an earache must choose between only a few options—prescribe an antihistamine, prescribe an antibiotic, perform surgery or do nothing. He looks in the ear, sees some redness and fluid, assumes there is a bacterial infection and prescribes an antibiotic. But, what has convinced him there are bacteria present?

Recall that harmful bacteria are *absent* in the middle ear fluid of about 30 to 50 percent of children with middle ear complaints. Dr. David P. Skoner reports that in children who have not responded to antibiotic therapy and tubes, the percentage of middle ears that contain *no harmful bacteria* is as high as 70 percent.[44]

The chances of inappropriate antibiotic prescribing are quite high when you consider the likelihood that no bacteria are present! Admittedly, middle ear cultures are difficult to perform unless the ear is draining because an incision (myringotomy) must be made in the eardrum to take a sample. Yet, not knowing the type of bacteria or its susceptibility to the chosen antibiotic can lead to choice of the wrong antibiotic. When no bacteria are present, antibiotic prescription is wholly inappropriate.

In one study, doctors were confronted with the case of a patient hospitalized for chronic bronchitis and pneumonia who was being treated with penicillin. They were also told the patient had a urinary tract infection confirmed by laboratory. When asked what they would do about it, *only 59 percent of physicians said they would recheck the urine to see if the infection had subsided.* Others said they would add other antibiotics to the therapy without a culture.[45]

Another recommendation in *The Physician's Desk Reference* reads as follows: "Prolonged use of X antibiotic may result in the overgrowth of nonsusceptible organisms."[46] Nonsusceptible organisms are those that are "supposed" to be susceptible to the antibiotic but have developed resistance, and those upon which the antibiotic normally has no effect—yeast, for example. Doctors should be aware of the ability of antibiotics to cause overgrowth of nonsusceptible organisms and take steps to minimize the impact. This was taken seriously years ago when many antibiotic preparations also contained substances to prevent the overgrowth of yeast. In the 1950s, physicians were advised to use acidophilus products such as Lactinex® (a product then from Parke Davis) when antibiotics were prescribed. Yet today, it seems to be given little consideration.

Science, Politics or Economics?

Contrary to popularly held beliefs, modern medicine is often based as much on philosophy, beliefs, politics and economics as it is on science. Perhaps no story better illustrates the tapestry interwoven by science, politics and economics than that of Dr. Erdem Cantekin, former director of a research center at the University of Pittsburgh. Dr. Cantekin, an international authority on ear disease, was co-investigator on a five-year National Institutes of Health study to evaluate the effectiveness of the antibiotic amoxicillin in the treatment of childrens' ear infections. Americans spend over $500 million annually to treat this one condition.

Cantekin's analysis of the data from this study showed that amoxicillin was ineffective and possibly harmful. His findings were further analyzed and corroborated by a statistical analyst from Carnegie Mellon University. But another researcher disagreed. According to an article entitled "Corporate-Funded Research May Be Hazardous to Your Health" published in the *Bulletin of the Atomic Scientist,* "the primary investigator on the $15 million federal grant, a colleague of Cantekin's at the medical school interpreted the data differently: *after changing the study protocol,* he determined that amoxicillin is effective against children's ear infections." [emphasis added]

"The primary investigator had also, over the period when the government was paying for the research, accepted perquisites amounting to over $50,000 per year in lecture fees and travel money from drug companies that produce antibiotics. Between 1981 and 1986, the ear center received more than $1.6 million in research grants from pharmaceutical companies to test the effectiveness of antibiotics on ear infections."

Dr. Cantekin wrote a paper arguing that amoxicillin "while appropriate for many uses, is not effective in the treatment of secretory otitis media [fluid behind the ear drum]." He submitted his paper for publication in hopes that other physicians could view his interpretation of the research and compare it with that of his colleague. But this was not to be. Both the *New England Journal of Medicine* and the *Journal of the American Medical Association* rejected Dr. Cantekin's paper. Meanwhile, the paper presented by his colleague, which supported antibiotic use, was published in the *New England Journal of Medicine* (1987). Antibiotic sales soared following publication of this paper.

This case is filled with tragic irony. As a result of Dr. Cantekin's efforts "his data tapes were erased, he was taken off all the department's grants, fired as director of the ear research clinic, and forbidden by the chairman to publish the paper. . . . Because he has tenure the School of Medicine cannot fire Cantekin, but he has been stripped of the resources needed to conduct research."[47,48] Sadly, as a result of these actions physicians throughout the United States were deprived of the opportunity to base their judgment on conflicting viewpoints, and were left to ponder only that which supported the prevailing belief.

Nearly five years later, Dr. Cantekin's paper was finally published in the *Journal of the American Medical Association* (December 1991). The results have seriously challenged the prevailing belief about the value of antibiotics in treating ear infections, especially those that are chronic. Cantekin's data showed that not only did children on amoxicillin fare no better than those taking placebo (sugar pill), but those on amoxicillin suffered from two to six times the rate of recurrent ear effusion. Cantekin also remarked on two other popular antibiotics. He wrote, ". . . those data indicate that amoxicillin was *not* effective and that two other antibiotics, Pediazole and cefaclor, also were *not* effective according to the method of analysis the OMRC [Otitis Media Research Center] had chosen to use."[49] It is interesting to note that the "negative" data regarding Pediazole and cefaclor was never published by the original investigators, but came out during a Congressional investigation.

Age- and Sex-Related Concerns

Concerns for the Elderly

The average age of Americans increases each year. For the next 50 years, the 85-and-older age group is expected to be the fastest-growing segment of the United States population. The number of people between the ages of 65 and 85 is expected to grow from 26 million to 30 million by the year 2000.[50]

According to a report in *Primary Care,* four out of five elderly persons have one or more chronic diseases. Conditions such as diabetes, atherosclerotic heart disease, chronic obstructive pulmonary disease and cerebrovascular disease may all predispose elderly people to infection. Older adults also are the most heavily medicated group of Americans. Drug therapy to treat chronic diseases may also increase the risk of infection. Many elderly people receive more than one drug. The average person over age 65 receives 10.7 prescriptions per year, compared with 4.3 for other age groups.[51] The risk of adverse drug reactions and risk of immune suppression go up with the number of drugs prescribed.

Elderly persons also have decreased kidney function. This makes prescribing of antibiotics, or any drug, a tricky matter. Medication can easily become toxic when kidney function is impaired. The most common infections in the elderly are pneumonia (which is the leading cause of death from an infectious disease in this age group), bronchitis, urinary tract infections, prostatitis and skin infections.[52] Diarrhea due to the bacterium *Clostridium dificile* is commonplace in hospitals and nursing homes (though by no means restricted to such places) largely because of the wide use of antibiotics. This bacteria can contribute to pseudomembranous colitis, a painful inflammatory condition of the bowel.[53]

Researchers believe that many of the immune problems associated with aging are due to poor nutritional status. In fact, poor nutrition is one of the most critical factors affecting infection susceptibility. People in nursing homes are at especially high risk for poor nutrition. When Dr. N.D. Penn and his co-workers supplemented elderly hospitalized patients with vitamins A, C and E, they noticed a significant improvement in immune function.[54] We also have noticed improved resistance to infection in elderly patients who have been placed on the proper diet with nutritional supplements. When one ages, the need for protein, fat and carbohydrate gradually goes down, but the need for vitamins and minerals generally does not.

One reason is that the ability to properly absorb nutrients decreases with age. A condition known as atrophic gastritis affects about 20 percent of people aged 60 to 69 and 40 percent of people over 80. This adversely influences the absorption of B_{12} and other nutrients. Elderly people are commonly deficient in B_6, B_2, vitamin C and vitamin D.

While important, vitamin and mineral supplements are not a panacea for the elderly. Vitamin A is not well-tolerated by some elderly people, especially if they have liver problems. In such cases, beta-carotene should be given. Also, elderly persons who take fish oils (EPA) for inflammatory or circulatory problems may be at risk to decreased immunity. The solution is to take extra vitamin E.

For you or an elderly family member in the hospital, nursing home or at home, you may wish to do the following:

- Have medications reviewed by an independent doctor. Often, one drug is given to treat the side effects of another drug. It is not uncommon for a person to have more than one doctor prescribe medication with none being aware of what the other is prescribing. This increases the risk of side effects and lowers immunity, increasing the risk of infection.

- Have an evaluation of nutritional status done by a clinical nutritionist or physician knowledgeable in clinical nutrition (an important distinction). Simple changes in diet can work wonders for health and immunity.

- Consider providing a nutritional supplement. A multivitamin is useful, but antioxidant nutrients such as vitamins C, E and beta-carotene are critical to immunity and to prevent some of the damage associated with aging.

- A supplement of acidophilus should be given whenever an elderly person is on antibiotics, and for three to four months thereafter. Acidophilus should also be considered if digestive problems such as irritable bowel syndrome or indigestion are present. These supplements are also important if a person has been treated with radiation or if they've had surgery.

Infants and Young Children

Antibiotic prescriptions to children under three have increased an incredible 51 percent over the past ten years.[55] It is in this age group that antibiotic overprescribing is most likely to occur. Middle ear problems account for roughly 42 percent of all antibiotics prescribed to children. Some doctors now wonder whether the misuse of antibiotics might actually be one cause of persistent earaches in children.

Recurrent earaches may be linked to hyperactivity as well. In one study, "69 percent of children evaluated for school failure who were receiving medication for hyperactivity gave a history of greater than 10 ear infections. By comparison, only 20 percent of non-hyperactive children had more than 10 infections."[56] Recurrent ear infections and hyperactivity have some common underlying dietary and nutritional features.

Dr. William Crook has long contended that there is a progression that begins with an upper respiratory infection or ear infection that is treated with antibiotics. This leads to overgrowth of yeast followed by more infections, which are then treated with more antibiotics. The yeast problem is aggravated, food allergies, earaches and behavior problems develop and the child is beset with recurrent infections for which antibiotics are again prescribed. This vicious cycle can repeat for months, even years!

Antibiotics have also been shown to contribute to bladder infections in children—even those with no history of bladder infections. In a study by Dr. K.J. Lidefelt, young girls treated with antibiotics for upper respiratory infections were found to develop subsequent bladder infections. This was believed to occur because the antibiotics suppressed one kind of bacteria while allowing another type to grow in the urethra and bladder.[57]

Many of the health problems of children aged zero to five years are related to food. Infants raised on formula are more prone to infections than those raised on breastmilk. Allergy or intolerance to food can lead to chronic mucus secretion in the middle ear, lungs, sinuses and nasal passages. The mucus-rich environment is ripe for the growth of bacteria, yeast and viruses. Any child who has persistent infections should be evaluated for food allergy or intolerance. Millions of children could avoid antibiotic exposure if such problems were addressed.

Nutrition also plays an important role in childhood illness. The dietary practices of today are vastly different from those of 50 years ago. Nutrient-depleted processed foods loaded with sugar and fat can make a child's smooth-running immune machinery turn into a "klunker." Nutrition is discussed later in this book.

For a discussion of diet, nutrition, allergy and earaches, see Dr. Schmidt's book *Childhood Ear Infections* and Dr. Smith's *Feed Your Kids Right.*

Women's Health

Women are among those most adversely affected by antibiotic use. They readily develop vaginal infections following antibiotic therapy. Bladder infection following antibiotic treatment for upper respiratory problems is also common. In some cases, vaginal infection causes a change in the acidity of the vagina, which sets the stage for bladder infections. Such women are caught in a vicious cycle of yeast infections and bladder infections. The antibiotics prescribed for bladder infection temporarily halt the illness, but it is followed by an aggravation of the vaginal infection. Women who have a history of bladder infections or yeast infections usually have deficiencies in the normal bacteria that live both in the intestines and the vagina. Supplementation by mouth with acidophilus (powder or capsules) and a vaginal douche used for several weeks (in severe cases, months) often solve this recurrent problem. Any woman who must take antibiotics should begin an oral supplement with acidophilus, and ask her doctor for a prescription of Nystatin to use as a douche ($\frac{1}{4}$ teaspoon Nystatin powder USP in 4 ounces of water) to prevent the vaginal yeast overgrowth. See Chapter 10 for more on this topic.

Many doctors fail to warn their female patients that antibiotics can interfere with the action of birth control pills. Numerous cases of pregnancy have occurred in women on oral contraceptives who took antibiotics with no knowledge of this effect.

Like any drug, antibiotics can cause problems when taken during pregnancy. Some antibiotics, such as tetracycline, have been shown to cause birth defects or miscarriage, especially when taken during the first trimester. Antibiotics are also readily passed into breastmilk. Thus, a lactating mother on antibiotics can pass a hefty dose of the drug to her nursing child. Whenever an antibiotic is prescribed during pregnancy or lactation, it is essential that women question the doctor about the necessity of such treatment.

Teenagers and Their Troubles

The teenage years seem to be a challenge to virtually everyone—the child, the parents, the school and society. We can add doctors to this list because the medical challenges of adolescence are formidable. Teenage acne is among them. It is estimated that up to 90 percent of teenagers will show some evidence of acne.[58] For this, physicians will prescribe substantial amounts of antibiotics, often keeping a child on them for years. The evidence that such antibiotics are effective for acne is not overwhelming, and many doctors believe that antibiotics used in this way contribute to ill health in teenagers. Dr. William G. Crook, pediatric allergist and author of numerous books on health and nutrition, believes the use of tetracycline and other antibiotics for acne is uncalled for. He states, "I've seen a number of patients with severe candida-related problems who gave a history of long-term tetracycline treatment for acne. . . . I now feel that routine use of tetracycline in managing teenage acne should be discontinued."[59]

Dietary and nutritional approaches to acne have been used with some success. It may be worthwhile to try the approach described in Chapter 10. Anyone who has been on antibiotics for acne should use an acidophilus supplement for several months to restore the normal balance of bacteria to the gut.

Teenage girls present another problem because many are becoming sexually active (obviously, boys are also). This increases the risk for bladder infections because intercourse is a common predisposing factor for bladder infections in females. Bladder infections are usually treated with antibiotics (although there are better means outlined in Chapter 10), but when treated in this way often give rise to vaginal yeast infections. Vaginal yeast infections present problems of their own. Both topics are discussed in Chapter 10.

In the Hospital

When people are hospitalized, they're often at their most vulnerable. They enter with an illness, are fearful and uncertain, will undergo invasive procedures, will receive medication and are exposed to countless varieties of germs. This puts the body at risk to developing a hospital-acquired infection. For these and other reasons, doctors are quick to put hospitalized patients on antibiotics. However, this does not always bode well for the patient.

One hospital study of antibiotic usage revealed that in 64 percent of the cases where antibiotics were involved, their use was either not indicated or they were improperly administered in terms of drugs or dosage.[60] The journal *Internal Medicine News* reported in 1983 that roughly 50 percent of surgeon-prescribed antibiotics are given when:[61]

- No infection is present.
- An incorrect drug is selected.
- A less expensive drug could have been selected.
- The dose is excessive.
- The duration of treatment or prophylaxis is excessive.

Surgeons often use antibiotics prophylactically in hopes of preventing the development of a postoperative infection. In most cases, the patient does not have an infection, but the doctor is "playing it safe." According to one study, 70.9 percent of such prescribing was considered "irrational on the basis of proved efficacy." Only 7.6 percent of antibiotics used in this manner was considered "rational."[62]

Hospitals have also become havens for bacteria that are resistant to antibiotics. We like to think of hospitals as sterile environments where hygiene and cleanliness are tightly controlled. Despite all the valiant efforts of hospitals to prevent the spread of infectious disease, germs run rampant. Many of these germs are highly resistant to antibiotics. Therefore, the germs have the potential to cause serious illness in hospitalized patients who are already immune-suppressed because of the debilitated states in which they find themselves. Who has not heard of someone who entered the hospital for "routine" surgery, but suffered a serious staph infection that required intravenous antibiotics and a lengthy stay.

According to Marti Kheel, when people enter the hospital they are at risk for *iatrogenic* (doctor-induced) disease. "Prescription drugs are causing more deaths each year than accidents on the road. . . . According to the FDA, 1.5 million Americans had to be hospitalized in 1978 as a consequence of taking prescription drugs. And some 30 percent of all hospitalized people get further damage by the therapy imposed upon them. The number of people killed in the U.S. by the intake of drugs has been estimated at 140,000 each year."[63]

It comes as no surprise that hospitalized patients are susceptible to nosocomial infections (those acquired in the hospital) when you consider their nutritional status. Some patients entering the hospital have disorders reflective of nutritional deficiency. If they have not entered with nutritional problems, they are likely to develop them during their stay. Dr. Joseph D. Beasley cites hospital studies in which 44 percent of general medical patients and as high as 50 percent of surgical patients suffered from protein-calorie malnutrition.[64] This does not include those with marginal, subclinical or single nutrient deficiencies. Optimal nutrition is a vital part of a healthy immune system. When nutritional status declines, susceptibility to infection increases. It seems negligent on the part of doctors and hospital staffs to prescribe volumes of antibiotics to hospitalized patients and pay no attention to nutrition—a factor so critical in boosting resistance to infections.

If you, a friend or a loved one is hospitalized for any reason, pay careful attention to nutritional status. Consuming red gelatin, mashed potatoes, white bread and cow's milk—common hospital fare—is no way to build immunity in a sick body. It is remarkable that nutritional supplements are so rarely given to hospital patients. In hospital situations where nutritional supplements have been prescribed, doctors have been able to prevent complications, speed recovery and manage infections. Unfortunately, such actions do not always sit well with the general hospital medical staff. As part of his routine surgical procedure, one physician customarily added a few grams of vitamin C to the intravenous fluids when putting in the closing stitches. The patients would awaken in 30 seconds and could walk back to the ward. This doctor was relieved of his hospital privileges for practicing this bit of "quackery."

At the Dentist

For many years it has been routine dental practice to treat all patients with a history of rheumatic fever, mitral valve prolapse or other such disorders with antibiotics. It was believed that streptococcal bacteria in the mouth could enter the bloodstream during routine dental procedures, such as cleaning teeth, and lodge themselves in the valves of the heart leading to a condition known as valvular endocarditis.

This practice exposes many thousands of patients to antibiotics each year who are not ill. It presents a special dilemma to patients who have yeast-related illness. Many suffer from mitral valve prolapse, a condition of the heart valve that puts them at "greater risk" for valve-related problems anyway. However, they also experience aggravation of their health when they are on antibiotics for any reason.

Physicians and dentists have followed the routine prescribing of antibiotics during dental work almost without question for some decades. It is interesting to note the contents of a paper entitled "Preventing Bacterial Endocarditis: A Statement for the Dental Profession," written by the Council on Dental Therapeutics of the American Heart Association. In this paper it states that, "Endocarditis may occur despite appropriate antibiotic prophylaxis. . . ." It also states, "Because no adequate, controlled clinical trials of antibiotic regimens for the prevention of bacterial endocarditis in humans have been done, recommendations are based on indirect information. . . ."[65]

A recent study conducted in the Netherlands attempted to assess the value of antibiotics used in this way. It has raised serious questions about whether the practice affords any benefit. The doctors found that in individuals undergoing a procedure for which preventive antibiotics were "indicated," there was little effect on the occurrence of endocarditis. Following the conclusion of this case-control study the investigators remarked that, in a country such as the Netherlands, complete compliance with endocarditis prophylaxis (prescribing preventive antibiotics during dental work to patients "at risk") would prevent only about *five* cases of the disease each year.[66]

Does this mean that dentists should no longer prescribe antibiotics for preventive purposes such as that described above? The American Dental Association and the American Heart Association are not likely to change their recommendations based on this one study. However, it is yet another study that raises questions about the way in which antibiotics are used and points to another area of possible antibiotic overuse.

According to Dwight Tschetter, D.D.S., a holistic dentist practicing in Minneapolis, the most frequently asked questions of holistic dentists are, "Are antibiotics necessary in my dental work?" and "Are there any alternatives to antibiotics?" Many patients seeking care from holistic dentists do not wish to receive antibiotics for routine dental procedures. Others have health conditions that are likely to be aggravated by antibiotics. Since prescribing antibiotics to "at risk" patients undergoing routine dental procedures is the *legal* standard of practice, all dentists are expected to comply—they are obligated to do it. If they do not comply, they risk losing their licenses or risk legal reprisal. Patients who choose not to use antibiotics during dental procedures do so at their own risk and are usually asked to sign a release stating that they choose not to use antibiotics and absolve the dentist of any liability should unforeseen consequences arise.

Patients and doctors who are concerned about this issue should obtain copies of the report by van der Meer entitled "Efficacy of Antibiotic Prophylaxis for Prevention of Native-valve Endocarditis." *Lancet* 1992;339:135–139, and "Preventing Bacterial Endocarditis: A Statement for the Dental Profession," Council on Dental Therapeutics, American Heart Association.

Doctor and Patient Attitudes

The doctor-patient relationship is distinct and unique. There are few relationships in which so much power and authority are given from one person to another. Each patient has his or her own personal relationship with a doctor, but there are certain expectations that are universal. One such expectation is that when you seek care from a doctor, he or she will "do something for you." Usually this means perform a procedure or prescribe a medication that might presumably solve your problem. You want to leave knowing someone understands what is going on in your body and that something is being done to correct the malady.

The dynamic of this relationship can have a significant impact on whether or not you receive treatment, and what kind of treatment that is. Doctors have a strong desire to determine what your problem is and then fix it. They also have a strong desire to please you by making you well and, no less important, perform well so they will retain you under their care. This can present a dilemma that can be characterized in the following example.

Imagine your child is feverish, coughing, irritable and has a runny nose. Although she is not seriously ill, you're concerned that she might become worse. You rush her to the pediatrician. Examination reveals some congestion in the lungs, a stuffed nose and a little redness of the eardrum. The temperature is 103 degrees fahrenheit. Whether it is due to a teething reaction, a virus or perhaps a bacterial infection of the middle ear, it is frightening. Your comfort zone is exceeded.

The doctor remarks, "Your daughter has some bronchial congestion and may be coming down with an ear infection." You reply, "Doctor, isn't there something you can do? I'm so worried about the coughing and waking at night. If she has an earache, won't she lose her hearing? Can't you give her something to make her more comfortable? I have to go to work in the morning and I won't sleep a wink!"

One of several things is occurring in this situation. The outcome will be based on the attitudes of both doctor and parent. If the doctor is one who prescribes antibiotics freely, he or she may simply say, "I'm going to write you a prescription for amoxicillin. Make sure you give it for the full 10 days. Also give your child some Tylenol to keep the fever down." If you are unquestioning, you will simply assume that the doctor knows "what's best" and follow the recommendations.

Alternatively, you might ask a series of questions about how the doctor arrived at this decision and whether your daughter is really sick enough to warrant the treatment. You may even question the doctor's judgment. Finally, you may waltz out the door, prescription in hand, feeling satisfied that "something" was done and that you've gotten your money's worth. Your day is saved!

The doctor who is more reluctant to write out the prescription may say, "Your daughter's fever isn't uncomfortably high, the ear congestion is slight, and the lung congestion isn't too bad. I would just like to wait and see if your daughter can beat this on her own."

This scenario also has several possibilities. The unquestioning parent will likely say, "I'm so glad to hear that she is not too ill." This mother will probably take her child home, watch her daughter improve, yet remain somewhat uncomfortable at her inability to facilitate her daughter's recovery. The next mother may inquire as to why the doctor decided as he did and ask if there are any other supportive things she can do. The third case involves the mother who is not satisfied with the result of this doctor visit. Her daughter is "sick" and "needs" treatment! This mother will not be satisfied until the doctor "does something!" In the third case, the mother may either overtly or covertly make her wishes known. In either case, the pressure will be on for the doctor to "come through," meaning to prescribe a drug.

Here is where the real dilemma arises. Many patients are dissatisfied if they leave the doctor's office without a treatment of some kind. They've just spent roughly 40 dollars on an office call and now they have to go back home and do what they were doing prior to the visit. These patients often place significant demands on their doctors to prescribe. They will often go elsewhere if the doctor does not comply with their wishes. In today's highly competitive world of medicine, the loss of any patient means a loss of revenue — perhaps even a temporary loss of esteem.

This side of doctors' behavior was made abundantly clear in a recent report by researchers at Harvard Medical School who studied the attitudes of doctors who were moderate to heavy prescribers of three drugs. According to a 1989 report in the *Wall Street Journal:* "Almost half the doctors said they were merely satisfying their patients' demands for these drugs and indicated fears that failure to meet such demands would risk losing patients to more obliging physicians. Many conceded that the prescribing couldn't be justified on scientific grounds. Another quarter of the doctors cited a 'placebo' effect as justification. Writing a prescription, they argued, can have a positive psychological benefit for the patients and thus possibly bring some relief."[67]

In one analysis published in the *New England Journal of Medicine,* doctors were presented with a hypothetical case in which a patient had been receiving procaine penicillin twice daily for pneumonia confirmed by blood culture. The patient demanded another drug when she still had a fever four days after the antibiotic had been started. Depending on their specialty, 29 to 47 percent of the doctors yielded to their patient's demands, even though the change in medication was not medically warranted.[68]

Pressure from a distraught patient is not good rationale for treatment of any kind. This is especially true with antibiotics, since the consequences can be far-reaching—especially in children.

Solution:

- Don't demand an antibiotic from your doctor. He or she may be uncertain of the need for an antibiotic. Your pressure may force him to choose that course when he might not otherwise do so. One of our colleagues in Minneapolis remarked, "My patients would be irate if I sent them out of here without an antibiotic." He admitted to often prescribing antibiotics, albeit reluctantly, to please his patients.

- Ask your doctor if there is anything that can be done short of giving an antibiotic. He may feel it is appropriate to wait a day or more, meanwhile using another means of treatment.

- Learn as many medical selfcare skills as possible about earaches, colds, sinus infections and other ailments.

Public Perception: The Myths of Antibiotic Use

Consumer demand is a powerful driving force in the world of medicine. When driven by inaccurate information, this demand can lead to inappropriate use of medical treatment. Over the years, many myths have emerged surrounding the application of antibiotics. In 1975, researchers at Mater Children's Hospital, South Brisbane, Australia asked 103 people a series of questions regarding antibiotic use. Their startling results are summarized below.[69]

What the public believed.

1. Antibiotics kill viruses.........................55%
2. Antibiotics kill bacteria.......................46%
3. Antibiotics are a stronger form of aspirin........13%

4. Penicillin is not an antibiotic.................... 15%

5. Antibiotics should be given for colds and flu..... 75%

6. Antibiotics should be given for gastroenteritis ... 40%

The responses given by those surveyed showed a remarkable degree of ignorance about antibiotics. One cannot expect laypersons to be educated to the extent of a physician. Yet, misconceptions about the usefulness of medical treatments make patients potential victims of improper care. The correct responses to the survey questions are given below.

1. No. Antibiotics *do not* kill viruses (or yeast). Viral infections are not helped by antibiotics.

2. Yes. Antibiotics kill bacteria. This is what they are designed for. That less than one half of those surveyed knew this is disconcerting.

3. No. Antibiotics kill bacteria; aspirin (and acetaminophen) combats fever and inflammation.

4. No. Penicillin is one of the most widely used antibiotics in the world.

5. No. Antibiotics should almost never be given for cold or flu because both conditions are due to viruses. Antibiotics are sometimes used when the flu becomes complicated by pneumonia.

6. No. Antibiotics should be used for gastroenteritis only when the cause is found to be bacterial by stool culture and testing.

Vast quantities of antibiotics are inappropriately given for viral and yeast infections. Since there is often confusion among the general public about what constitutes these and other microorganisms, let us define them briefly here. Bacteria are one-celled living things. They have their own metabolism and can live outside of living cells. Staph and strep are examples of bacteria. In contrast, viruses are not living. They are more like pieces of genetic material (DNA or RNA) surrounded by a coat of protein. Viruses must live inside a living cell in order to survive and reproduce. The common cold, flu, herpes and measles are caused by viruses. Yeast are single-celled creatures that belong to the plant kingdom. They are cousins to the molds you find in your damp basement or on old bread. There are many classes of yeast including that in brewer's and baker's yeast. One type, *Candida albicans,* accounts for much human illness.

But Doctor, Are You Sure?

Medicine is both an art and a science. It is not exact. The standing joke among doctors—"Why do you think they call it medical *practice?"*—reflects this. While medicine is constantly evolving in an attempt to be more accurate in diagnosis and treatment, there is sometimes substantial room for error. This can have chilling implications, especially when the treatment prescribed is not without harm. We would like our doctors to be sure of their assessment of our health—for example, that an infection is present and an antibiotic is needed. However, they are often limited by beliefs, time, technology and a host of other factors.

In one study, to assess the diagnostic accuracy of physicians, 10 board-certified or board-eligible medical school faculty members were asked to examine 308 patients who complained of sore throat. The doctors were to estimate the probability of these patients having strep throat and reveal what form of treatment they would recommend. Treatment was to be recommended before laboratory results were known, as is commonly done in private practice.

These experienced and highly trained physicians estimated that 81 percent of the patients had strep throat. In reality, only 4.9 percent were found to have positive cultures for strep after laboratory analysis. Perhaps most alarming was the fact that 104 of the 308 patients were actually started on antibiotic therapy. Only eight of the patients required antibiotics. According to the researchers, "If overtreatment is defined as the use of antibiotics in culture-negative patients, the physicians' probability overestimation was associated with substantial overtreatment."[70,71]

This phenomenon appears not to be limited to just one group of doctors in one study. In a recent study (1989) of 222 people with sore throat, doctors believed that 50.5 percent had strep infections. However, culture results showed that only 13.5 percent were positive for strep. Most of these patients would have been given antibiotics needlessly.[72]

This phenomenon is surprising when you consider the view expressed in the textbook *Infections: Recognition, Understanding, Treatment,* which states "Pharyngitis and tonsillitis affect many people each year and have a considerable socioeconomic impact. These disorders are the most common reasons for consulting a physician. Unfortunately, however, *they are also among the worst treated of all illnesses, primarily because of the overprescription of antibiotics."* [emphasis added][73]

Antibiotics are commonly used in the treatment of fever, based on the belief that fever is often due to bacterial infection. Dr. David M. Jaffe studied the course of high fever in 955 children under 3 who were treated at hospital emergency rooms. He wondered if antibiotics should be given routinely in such cases. One half of the children were given amoxicillin while the other half received a placebo. Dr. Jaffe found that there was virtually *no difference in fever outcome* in antibiotic-treated children when compared with those given the placebo. Only a few children, who were later found to have bacterial infection, responded to amoxicillin. Dr. Jaffe concluded that antibiotics are "not advisable" for most children with high fever.[74] This study is somewhat alarming. Antibiotics were *given needlessly in over 90 percent* of these children with fever. What effect might this have on their health? In how many emergency rooms across the U.S., Canada and Europe are antibiotics used in this way?

There are other such accounts of mistakes in judgment that have resulted in overuse of antibiotics. These are but a few that serve to remind us that doctors do not have all the answers; they are not always right. They are, in fact, very often wrong. This should send a signal that we must each be the guardian of our own and our children's health. Be an informed consumer of health care. Become an activated patient (described in Chapter 10). Ask questions. Enter into a health partnership with your doctor rather than surrender your control to the doctor.

Doctors Are Different

In our world of high-tech medicine and standardized medical training, we would like to believe that one doctor will treat a problem much like the next doctor. However, anyone who has sought a second or third opinion for a health problem knows that disagreement among doctors is often the rule rather than the exception. Finding doctors who agree is sometimes like asking a Republican or a Democrat which is the best solution for balancing the budget! Personal opinion, philosophy, belief systems, and even case load are important determinants, as illustrated by the following classic study of physician judgment.

Doctors were asked their opinion on the need for tonsillectomy in 1,000 children. The author reported, "Of these [1,000 children], some 611 had had their tonsils removed. The remaining 389 were examined by other physicians, and 174 were selected for tonsillectomy. This left 215 children whose tonsils were apparently normal. Another group of doctors was put to work examining these 215 children, and 99 of them were adjudged in need of tonsillectomy. Still another group of doctors was then employed to examine the remaining children, and nearly one half were recommended for the operation."[75] Were all these tonsillectomies necessary? On what basis did one group of doctors decide tonsillectomy was not needed while another group believed surgery was indicated? It becomes obvious from such a study that there is a strong degree of personal opinion and bias involved when doctors decide which procedures are needed.

Doctors also vary regarding their basic medical knowledge. Knowledge about proper use of antibiotics is no exception. In a recent issue of *Pediatrics,* F. A. Disney, M.D., former president of the American Board of Pediatrics, discussed a telephone conference dealing with the choice and use of antibiotics. Disney remarked that he was "astonished" and "alarmed" at the methods that certified pediatricians in practice were using to select antibiotics. Most disconcerting were assertions that the antibiotic was commonly "picked at random or was selected by the doctor's preference for one drug or another chosen on the basis of available samples or side effects . . ." One doctor stated that "if the child wasn't better by the end of a period of time, then all drugs were stopped and subsequently the child sometimes did recover." Dr. Disney suggested that in such cases "possibly the drugs were contributing to the child's illness."[76]

Are Antibiotics the Best Medicine?

In 1975, a televised "National Antibiotic Therapy Test" was held in the United States to assess doctors' knowledge in the use of antibiotics in treating infectious disease. A total of 4,500 medical specialists participated in the test. Cases were presented that simulated real-life clinical problems a doctor might encounter in daily practice. Doctors were then asked about appropriate treatment.

The results can only be described as frightening when one considers the extent to which antibiotics are prescribed. Only *two* doctors out of 4,500 received perfect scores. Researchers analyzed the results to determine which doctors scored above 80 percent (below 75 percent is a failing grade on most medical school, graduate school and state medical board examinations). The results were further broken down by specialty. The percentage of doctors in each specialty who scored above 80 percent is shown below:[77]

Surgeons	10%
Family practitioners	15%
Ob/Gyn	18%
Pediatricians	24%
Internists	38%
Infectious disease experts	83%

Doctors who had been in practice the longest (>15 years) received the lowest scores, as did those who saw the most patients per day (>30 patients). Are the results of this study reflective of the average doctor in practice? It is difficult to know. But this study seems to raise serious questions about antibiotic use and whether most doctors are appropriately equipped to deal with the complexities of antibiotic therapy.

One medical analyst noted that "the majority [of doctors] displayed a potentially dangerous degree of ignorance."[78,79] That most doctors displayed this degree of ignorance about antibiotics is itself frightening. That the busiest doctors tended to score the worst does not bode well for patients who must seek care from already overworked doctors. Doctors who see more patients per hour are more likely to be poor prescribers, use drugs inappropriately more often, and do incomplete physical exams.[80] This commonly results in more adverse drug side effects because the drug was either not needed or incorrectly chosen. It also frequently leads to more patient visits because the patient's original problem was not solved. According to pharmacologist Arabella Melville, Ph.D., "These physicians set up a vicious circle, creating a heavier workload, which in turn leads to higher prescribing and increased risk because non-pharmacological options become more remote."[81]

Doctors Are Not Taught About Alternatives in Medical School

A basic tenet of allopathic medicine is that infections are due to organisms (bacteria, viruses or parasites). Organisms can be killed with antibiotics. Therefore, infections should be treated with antibiotics. This view has changed little during the past fifty years despite evidence that the underlying theory is fragmentary and insufficient to explain why we succumb to these organisms.

Antibiotics are usually chosen without regard to factors such as diet and nutrition. This is remarkable when you consider that deficiency of key nutrients has a substantial impact on our resistance to infection. For example, deficiency of zinc and vitamin A can increase susceptibility to infection by bacteria and viruses. Disregard of nutritional factors is even more surprising in light of evidence that infection itself can *cause* nutrient deficiencies that further hinder our infection-fighting capabilities.

There has been a virtual explosion of information about clinical nutrition in the scientific literature over the past decade. The general public often believes that their physician has kept abreast of these breakthroughs and has considered nutritional therapy in the course of treating their patients. The sad reality, however, is quite different. In 1986, the Food and Nutrition Board of the National Academy of Sciences concluded that "nutrition education programs in U.S. medical schools are largely inadequate to meet the demands of the medical profession." The committee also found that "nutrition is seldom taught as a separate course . . ." and that there are an "insufficient number of hours devoted to nutrition and inconsistency in the scope and depth of topics."[82]

Medical doctors receive almost no training in nutrition. In medical schools where nutrition is offered, it is usually offered as an elective course. In 1991, Dr. Sehnert spoke to a medical resident while returning home on a flight from San Diego. When Sehnert asked the young doctor how much training he had received in nutrition, the reply was, "We had an eight-hour elective in nutrition, but most people didn't take it." He went on to say that the University of Illinois Medical School, where he was a student, had one of the better programs.

Medical licensing exams do not even test specifically in the area of clinical nutrition. Unless the individual doctor takes the initiative, he or she is not likely to learn about nutrition or utilize it in practice. Thus, when you seek care for illness, your treatment options are often limited to drugs.

Several years ago, one of Ralph Nader's organizations, the Center for Science in the Public Interest, which publishes the monthly *Nutrition Action,* conducted an unusual survey. They gave a basic nutrition quiz to two groups of people—M.D.s and their receptionists. The results were shocking if not alarming. Nearly all the receptionists passed with flying colors. We won't mention who flunked most of the time!

Reliance upon drugs as the backbone of therapy causes doctors to overlook viable alternatives that may help their patients who suffer not only from infections, but illness of all types. Consider the following discoveries about non-antibiotic approaches to infection that have been reported in scientific studies:

- The plant *Lentinus edodes* has been shown in numerous trials to inhibit the replication of viruses and slow the progress of viral infections.

- *Hypericum triquetrifolium,* better known as St. John's Wort, prevents the growth and infectivity of viruses.

- Extracts of the herb *Echinacea* have been used by European doctors to successfully treat infections of the upper respiratory tract, including whooping cough, bronchitis and tonsillitis.

- Intravenous doses of vitamin C have been used to successfully treat meningitis, pneumonia and other infections.

- Oil of *Melaleuca alternifolia,* or tea tree oil, has some of the widest-ranging antimicrobial properties of any plant.

- Vitamin A has been used to reduce the rate of pneumonia and croup in children suffering from severe measles.

- The juices of blueberry and cranberry have been shown in university trials to be effective in the treatment of bladder infections in women, even in cases involving antibiotic-resistant bacteria.

All of this work is published in the medical literature! (It will be discussed in more detail in later chapters of this book.) If doctors had training in the use of these alternatives, we would be able to sharply reduce the use of antibiotics and the untoward effects that often follow.

Are Antibiotics Being Overused in Your Care?

Doctors usually prescribe antibiotics with sincere motives. That is, they hope the antibiotic will help their patients get well and prevent complications. Obviously, no doctor sets out to intentionally harm patients. Yet doctors have different comfort zones with respect to antibiotics. Some doctors use antibiotics with full awareness of the consequences and restrict their use to only clear indications. Other doctors are somewhat cautious yet quite confident that antibiotics are the solution—thus prescribing somewhat liberally. Others prescribe antibiotics in an almost knee-jerk fashion, giving them at the mere hint of something wrong.

The following guidelines will help you decide if your doctor might be prescribing antibiotics too liberally. Place a "1" next to each item that applies.

____ Prescribes antibiotics over the phone.

____ Grants a refill of an antibiotic prescription without seeing you or your child.

____ Prescribes antibiotics to a child who is relatively healthy.

____ Prescribes antibiotics without at least ordering a differential blood count.

53

_____ Prescribes antibiotics without addressing your diet and nutritional status.

_____ Prescribes antibiotics after only a brief or cursory examination.

_____ Seems to ignore or "write off" your descriptions of antibiotic reactions in you or your child.

_____ Remarks to you that antibiotics are harmless and cause no side effects.

_____ Does not take your concerns about antibiotic safety seriously.

_____ Has prescribed several courses of one or more antibiotics without improvement in you or your child, and simply proceeds to prescribe another antibiotic.

_____ Prescribes antibiotics when there are clear indications the illness is viral in origin (for instance, a cold).

_____ Prescribes antibiotics without doing a culture.

_____ Does your doctor seem overworked or overbooked?

_____ Does he/she tend to cut your visit short by handing you a prescription and walking out the door?

_____ Total

If the total score is more than 5 you may be receiving antibiotics needlessly. One solution is to bring your concerns to the attention of your doctor. Ask for a full re-evaluation of the situation. If you are not comfortable with your progress, seek another opinion.

One patient, upon bringing her concerns about antibiotic safety to her doctor's attention, was confronted with a gruff "what medical school did you go to?" Could this doctor be seriously concerned about his patient's welfare? It seems that in such circumstances, we believe, a change of doctor is in order.

Why Use Antibiotics?

Does this mounting evidence against antibiotics suggest their use be discontinued? The answer is an obvious "no." But we must draw a distinction between appropriate use and overuse. As we stated earlier, many lives have been saved by the prudent use of antibiotics. There are many circumstances in which antibiotics have been the deciding factor over whether the patient remained in the here-and-now or moved on to the "Hereafter." People get sick with infections that overwhelm them for one reason or another. Master puppeteer Jim Henson died of acute pneumonia. One day he was fine, the next day he checked into the hospital, the next day he died. Jim Henson needed heroics, he needed antibiotics, as do many others.

There are two important considerations in the use of antibiotics: whether an infection is acute or chronic, and whether the person's immune system is compromised such as in AIDS. In acute infections, or those that come on rapidly with severe symptoms, antibiotics seem more justified, provided the correct diagnosis is made. In chronic infections where antibiotics have been used repeatedly with minimal success, the use of antibiotics is more questionable. In immune-compromised individuals, antibiotics are perhaps necessary to treat opportunistic infections, but such people also need tremendous support in the way of diet, nutrition, social and psychological help and lifestyle changes.

Many of the problems described in this chapter could be avoided or minimized if doctors adopted some of the following guidelines:

1. Limit the number of antibiotics in use. In the U.S. some 3,000 antibiotics are available for doctors to use. In some European countries, the authorities restrict the use of many antibiotics. This ensures that there will always be antibiotics available should life-threatening bacteria be resistant to the antibiotics currently in use.

2. Always perform cultures to determine if bacteria are present and which type of bacteria are present.

3. Perform susceptibility tests to identify the antibiotic that will be most effective against the bacteria in question.

4. Use the antibiotic with the narrowest spectrum of action. This minimizes the negative effects on normal body bacteria and optimizes the effect on the infecting bacteria.

5. Avoid broad-spectrum antibiotics when possible. They wipe out nearly everything in their path. Examples include Keflex, Bactrim, Septra, ampicillin, Ceclor and amoxicillin. William Crook, M.D. states, "If I feel an antibiotic is indicated in treating a respiratory or skin infection, I nearly always first use penicillin V, penicillin G or erythromycin. These antibiotics do not wipe out the normal intestinal flora, which encourages the growth of Candida albicans."[83]

6. Prescribe a short course of the antifungal drug nystatin. According to Dr. Crook, "If I prescribe a broad-spectrum antibiotic, I always give nystatin along with the antibiotic to discourage yeast overgrowth."[84] Dr. Crook's recommendation that nystatin be given along with the antibiotic is offered by many physicians concerned about antibiotic side effects. When your doctor prescribes a broad-spectrum antibiotic ask if he or she will also prescribe a short course of nystatin.

7. Prescribe antibiotics for the shortest possible duration. Some studies have shown two-, three-, five- and seven-day courses to be as effective as ten-day courses (for ear infections). It has also been shown that 500 mg of vitamin C given with every 250 mg of tetracycline increased the blood level of the antibiotic 15-fold compared with tetracycline alone. Such an approach (providing antibiotics are needed) could reduce the amount of antibiotic given and shorten the course of antibiotic therapy, thus minimizing the side effects.[85]

8. Always recommend acidophilus for adults or bifidus for children under five whenever antibiotics are taken. This will help prevent yeast infection, intestinal upset and food allergy/intolerance.

9. Always try to identify the underlying reasons why the patient became ill. Consider diet, nutrition, lifestyle, hygiene, stress and environmental factors.

10. Always recommend nutritional supplements during times of infection.

11. Consider the use of homeopathic or botanical medicine along with antibiotic therapy.

Only your doctor can make the precise determination of whether an antibiotic is needed and which antibiotic is best in a given situation. In our view, **antibiotics should never be used alone.** They should always be used in conjunction with methods that boost immunity and improve resistance! These are what we call the healthier options for families, and are described throughout the remainder of this book.

II

Why We Get Sick

3

The Miracle of Immunity

"We have given too much attention to the enemy and have to some extent overlooked our defenses."

M. Behar
World Health Organization[1]

The amazing immune system we each possess is not only priceless and complex, it makes possible what all of us have in common. We may be different in gender, color of hair and skin, religion and job. But we have a common bond—we are all survivors. Our parents survived long enough to conceive us. Grandparents had the same claim for your parents. The thing that made this possible is that precious commodity—the immune system. With it functioning well, one has good health. Without proper functioning, one simply can't survive!

Your immune system does much more than help you recover from a cold or the flu or the chicken pox. It is an awesome network that involves defender cells and lymph nodes and bone marrow. It is more than a bunch of "PAC-man" cells that gobble up viruses, bacteria, yeasts and other invaders. It could be described as a sophisticated storm warning weather service/strategic air command-national guard/garbage collection-clean-up service/antibody manufacturing-storage company/delivery and information network.

It has been said that to learn humans seem to need the "three Ms: Misery, Murder and Mayhem." That seems to be the case regarding many of our major breakthroughs in science and health.

It took the misery of World War I to develop antisepsis and the improved techniques of modern surgery. It took World War II and the Japanese prison camps of Singapore to demonstrate that malnutrition can cause schizophrenic-type mental disorders that can be reversed by nutritional means. It took the mayhem of today's AIDS epidemic to show us some of the insights we now have concerning our amazing immune system.

This system has a complex assignment: locate and destroy all substances, living or inert, not properly part of your human body. It has the miraculous ability to sort substances that you breathe, drink or ingest into two classes: "self" or "not self"—or in other words, "friend" or "foe."

This complex task is accomplished in orderly phases, some well but others poorly understood. These have now been described in hundreds of articles and scores of books. Each response is determined by the nature of the foe. There is one response to pathogens such as viruses, bacteria, protozoa or yeasts like *Candida albicans.* There is another response to substances like alcohol, nicotine, marijuana or cocaine. There is still another to the environmental toxins so common in today's world—car exhaust, pesticides, paint fumes or substances such as asbestos fibers. In many people even common foods like milk/dairy products, chocolate, wheat and corn can cause immune reactions. And, finally, there are the everyday reactions to ragweed, dusts, pollens and molds that can plague so many of us.

The immune response may last only a few minutes if you inhale a small puff of ragweed dust, or months for some bacteria or parasites. Some symptoms may be obvious like a headache or skin rash. Others may be much harder to spot, with general symptoms such as fatigue, frequent infections or loss of stamina. When patients go to their doctor and say, "Doctor, I'm tired all the time" or "I just don't have the strength I used to have," a physician can be perplexed about what to check or what to advise.

While these puzzling symptoms are being played out, the "war within" is being fought. The white cells (one trillion strong) are banded together to do "battle." An excellent description of this "army" of defenders was presented not in a medical journal, but in the June 1986 *National Geographic.*[2]

The Miracle of Immunity

This excellent article, "The Wars Within," by Peter Jaret and Steven B. Mizel described the components of the immune system using military terms:*

Macrophages—"Frontline defender" and housekeeper, these cells digest debris in the bloodstream with a PAC-man-like maneuver when they encounter a foreign organism (virus, bacteria, yeast, etc.).

Helper T-cells—As "army generals," these cells direct the immune system. They identify the "enemy" and then rush to the spleen and lymph nodes. There they stimulate the production of other cells to fight the infection. Called T-cells (or thymus cells), they originate in the thymus gland, the "West Point Academy" of the immune system. The thymus is located in the chest between the sternum (breast bone) and the heart.

Killer T-cells—"Recruited" and activated by helper T-cells, these specialists kill the cells (mucous cells of the lungs or throat, for example) that have been invaded by outside organisms. They also destroy cells that have turned cancerous.

B-cells—These cells are an "arms factory" that reside in the spleen (an organ in the upper left part of the abdomen under the ribs) or the lymph nodes. They are induced by the helper T-cells to produce antibodies.

Antibodies—These protein molecules are manufactured by the B-cells and target specific "invaders." They are rushed to the

---

*The military analogy is used here because many facets of the immune response can be easily described in military terms, terms that are familiar to many readers. However, a growing number of researchers are uncomfortable with the military analogy, preferring one that is more harmonious. Doctors working with seriously ill patients, using guided imagery to help boost immune function, find that visualizing the immune system in violent or military terms is less successful than viewing it in more harmonious terms. We wholeheartedly agree in theory and in practice. For example, psychologist Stephen Levine reports on a woman who overcame her cancer only after switching from battlefield imagery (sending heavily armed soldiers) to sending loving troubadours to "caress and massage and sing and tickle my tumors away."[3] Still, for the purposes of illustration and simplicity, we have employed the more commonly used military analogy here.

"front line" where they neutralize the enemy or tag it in some way for attack by other cells.

Suppressor T-cells—This third type of T-cell, also a "graduate of West Point," is able to slow down or stop the activity of the B-cells and other T-cells. They call off the "attack" after the acute phase of the infection while the body goes into the convalescent or recovery phase.

Memory cells—These cells are generated by the initial infection and may circulate in the blood or lymph for years. Some give lifelong immunity to you after the initial infection of, for example, chickenpox. They enable the body to respond quickly to subsequent invasions of that virus.

Using more military terms, here is a summary of what happens. When a flu virus arrives in your body by way of droplets in a sneeze or direct contact with your hands, the scene is set for the cell wars.

1. The "battle" begins—As the virus invades your body, the first few are given the PAC-man treatment by "sentry dog" macrophages, which seize the virus's antigens (toxins) and gobble them up. Some cells display this event on their own surface like a neon "help wanted" sign. Among frontline defender cells, a select few are programmed to "read" these neon signs. They bind themselves to the macrophage cell. Other helper T-cells "seeing" this take place rush to the spleen and lymph nodes for more help.

2. The forces multiply—With this "red alert" from the helper T-cells, there is a "mobilization of the National Guard" back home in the lymphatic system. Next, there is a multiplication of killer T-cells, which start arriving at the "front lines." The B-cells, the tiny arms factories described earlier, start production of antibodies. An "airlift" of these supplies then begins.

3. Conquering the infection—As the invasion of the virus continues more trouble occurs, especially if the host has its defenses down because of stress overload, poor nutrition, faulty lifestyles, etc. This happens as a few of the viruses

begin to enter the inside of cells. There they unite with
the DNA in the nucleus and begin to replicate and
multiply. They steal nourishment at the cellular level, and
a miniature virus factory is started. Killer T-cells that
arrive on the scene must first destroy the body's own cells.
This is done by chemically puncturing their membranes.
This in turn lets the viral contents spill out and disrupts
viral multiplication. Antibodies have by this time arrived
to neutralize the viruses and clump around the viral
surfaces to prevent them from attacking other cells.

4. Calling a truce—As the infection becomes confined to a
part of your body, for example a carbuncle on your leg or
a crypt in your tonsil, the "headquarters battalion" in the
thymus sends out suppressor T-cells to slow down the
immune response. Memory cells (the "Intelligence
Corps") make notes called cellular memory that can then
quickly respond the next time some virus shows up to try
to make trouble.

It should be noted here that not only do the memory cells make
notes about what happened, but on the other side of the fight,
some of the virus enemies do the same evolving devious methods to
sabotage and escape detection. The viruses that cause influenza
may mutate and change their "fingerprints." (Examples of this are
the Asian flu and Hong Kong flu.) The AIDS virus is one of the
most crafty of all and can hide for months in healthy cells. In some
cases this deadly virus short-circuits the entire immune process
and eventually kills its host.

This ability to short-circuit the immune system is also true of
the yeast *Candida albicans*—the culprit candida-related complex
(CRC) or systemic candidiasis. Researcher David Soll of the University of Iowa has documented that *Candida albicans* and several
of its yeast "cousins" are capable of gene jumping and not only
switching forms but colony shapes. Soll and his co-workers have
called this fungus a "maddening Jekyll-Hyde yeast" because of
this tactic it uses for survival.[4]

Integral to all the activity noted above are several chemical
messenger services. The "Signal Corps" has protein messengers
that have these mind-boggling biochemical names:

1. Interleukin-1—This is secreted by the macrophage and signals or activates helper T-cells. These then rush back to the spleen and lymph nodes to get white blood cell production going.

2. Interleukin-2—Activated T-cells produce this lymphokine messenger to stimulate production of other helper cells and killer T-cells.

3. B-cell growth factor—This is also secreted by T-cells to make B-cells stop replicating and start making antibodies.

4. Gamma interferon—Made by helper T-cells, it activates killer T-cells and enables them to attack the invading organisms. It also affects macrophages, keeping them at the site of the infection and helping them digest the invaders they have trapped.

With this insight into how your amazing immune system works, the next question that comes to mind is why *doesn't* it work some-times? Why can people go for years and have no trouble, and all of a sudden they are "allergic" to peanuts or chocolate or sunflower seeds? Why are some people driven beyond the borders of physi-ological tolerance by certain stressors? Are viral, bacterial or can-dida infections causative or opportunistic? In other words, do they *cause* trouble alone or do they seize the *opportunity* to invade when your defenses are down for one reason or another?

Whoever provides the answer will likely go directly to Stock-holm to pick up the Nobel Prize for Medicine. The reality is that we still don't know. There are, however, some common roots. Some of these are specific while others are more general. Most sources of illness involve one or more of these Five Vital Factors:

1. Excessive antibiotics—As explained previously, since the introduction of broad spectrum antibiotics in the 1950s— both in medical and veterinary use—bacterial resistance and other problems related to antibiotic abuse have become far too common. The normal balance of essential microflora has been disturbed in some people by excessive use of antibiotics which kill not only the "bad guys" but also the "good guys" such as *Lactobacillus acidophilus,* a friendly bacteria needed for proper digestion.

2. Food and nutrition—Whether it's the Alar on apples, the yellow dye #5 in certain foods, the MSG in the Chinese soup, the lead, pesticides and chlorine in our tap water, or whatever, these foreign substances take their toll on one's immunity. The amount of "anti-nutrients," or substances that antagonize nutrients in our bodies, has increased dramatically over the past 50 years. As we eat more calorie-rich, nutrient-poor, refined food, the nutrients needed for proper immunity become less available to us.

3. Environment—The damage to our environment, whether it's the Exxon oil spill in Alaska, the acid rain in Vermont or Quebec, the Love Canal damage in New York or smog in California, takes its toll both without and within our bodies. Each day we are being exposed to more and more synthetic chemicals. Together, they exert a cumulative effect that puts a heavy load on an immune system already taxed by the complexities of the twentieth century.

4. Heredity, lifestyle and hygiene—The lifestyle changes of the past 50 years have been striking. We work longer hours, have less time for leisure, exercise less, watch more TV, sleep less, have more sleep disorders, spend less time outdoors with nature and fresh air, and on and on. Our lifestyle and habits have a profound effect on our immune system and resistance to disease. With the social changes of the last 25 years has come greater use of not just the illegal drugs (cocaine, marijuana and crack) but also the legal drugs (alcohol, nicotine, caffeine). These chemicals are all viewed by the immune system as foes and must be detoxified. This makes extra demands on the immune system and can wear it down.

   Our individual genetic tendencies influence how we respond to the varied stresses present in our environment.

5. Mood, mind and stress—These days we are all experiencing more types and larger episodes of stress that affect us in many ways. For some it is caused by divorce, others by mobility and still others by the great number of changes we make through different homes, new jobs, and

so on. There is more depression and stress-related disability than at any time in our history. Most of us experience much more such stress than did our parents or grandparents. Stress can cause the immune system to come "unglued."

The immune system will function best when we consider the Five Vital Factors, remove or minimize those factors that are harmful, and utilize or optimize those that are beneficial. It is not complicated. It is based on common sense, moderation and balance. In fact, balance may be the most important part of building a healthy immune system. Balancing the Five Vital Factors is the focus of the next four chapters.

4

Food, Nutrition and Infection Susceptibility

"There is no longer reason to doubt that nutritional status does influence the course of infectious disease in man and animals."

Drs. Paul M. Newberne and Gail Williams
Massachusetts Institute of Technology[1]

"The best vaccine against common infectious diseases is an adequate diet."

World Health Organization[2]

Carol was a 35-year-old woman with a degree in nutrition science. She suffered from severe chronic fatigue, recurrent vaginal infections, recurrent bladder infections and recurrent upper respiratory infections. For years she was on antibiotics on a regular basis. After treatment of a respiratory infection, she developed a bladder infection. Once the bladder infection was resolved, she developed tonsillitis. She suffered from chronic sinus pain and postnasal drip. Each new year was accompanied by a roller coaster of infections and antibiotics. Despite all the antibiotic prescriptions by the best doctors in town, Carol did not improve. It seemed as though there was no solution in sight.

Carol had reached the limits of her tolerance. She finally realized that she was continually sick for a reason—a reason that was not being addressed by antibiotic therapy. She wanted a change in medical philosophy, which brought her to the office of Dr. Schmidt. Schmidt took a close look at Carol's diet and history. When Carol revealed she was a food tester for a large Midwest food manufacturer, a "red flag" went up. This began to look like a food allergy problem. Then she specified she was a food "taster" in the dairy division. Essentially, she spent her days at work tasting specialty foods that contained dairy products—all day long, day after day, month after month, year after year. It appeared as though Carol's body was so burdened by the high daily doses of dairy products that her immune system went on the blink.

Food elimination tests and blood tests revealed that Carol was extremely allergic to dairy products. She took a three-month medical leave during which she avoided dairy products entirely. Gradually her immune system began to respond. The respiratory and bladder infections she had at the time of her first visit improved without antibiotics. After the elimination of dairy-containing foods, her recurrent infections ceased.

After many months of markedly improved health, Carol drank a cup of cow's milk. Within 24 hours, she developed a high fever, tonsillitis and a deep cough. Many symptoms persisted for two months after this exposure. These were some of the same symptoms from which she suffered before. She was indeed sensitive to cow's milk and the "challenge" confirmed it.

This is just one example of the way food can affect immunity and infection susceptibility. Doctors have known for centuries that nutrition is one of the greatest influences on our resistance to all disease.

How Nutrition Affects Immunity and Infection Susceptibility

Nutritional deficiency comes in all shapes and sizes. General malnutrition as seen commonly in Third World countries is a well-known example. Infection is a major killer of children in these countries. Diseases such as measles, which is rarely fatal in the West, are a common cause of death among the malnourished.

According to Bernard Dixon, Ph.D., author of *Beyond the Magic Bullet,* nutrition can influence infection in a two-way interaction. Nutritional deficiency makes it easier for organisms to invade the body and establish themselves. It also slows recovery and convalescence from illness.[3] In addition, infection adversely affects nutritional status in several ways. First, infection may impair appetite and absorption, thus limiting the amount of nutrients available to the body. Second, the presence of bacteria or viruses may cause the body to rapidly use its stores of nutrients such as vitamin C and zinc, and may cause vitamin A to be used up faster than it can be mobilized from the liver stores.

In 1970, Drs. Paul Newberne and Gail Williams, then at the Massachusetts Institute of Technology, contributed to a book entitled *Nutritional Influences in the Cause of Infectious Disease*. They describe four important ways in which nutrition can influence infection. Nutritional deficiency can:[4]

1. Adversely affect the body, which makes it easier for the bacteria or virus to invade.
2. Have an effect on the bacteria or virus once it has established itself in the body.
3. Increase susceptibility to secondary infection.
4. Retard convalescence after infection.

Physician and researcher Thomas McKeown has spent considerable time investigating the underlying reasons humans become ill. He states that "the relationship [between man and microorganism] is stable and finely balanced according to the physiological states of the host and parasite; an improvement in nutrition would tip the balance in favor of the former, and a deterioration in favor of the latter."[5] McKeown further states, "A severe degree of deficiency of almost any of the essential nutrients may have a marked effect on the manner in which the host responds to an infectious agent. The same infection may be mild or even unapparent in a well-nourished host, but virulent and sometimes fatal in one that is malnourished."[6]

There is growing evidence that vitamin and mineral deficiency can lead to diminished immunity and increased infection susceptibility, and that supplementation can boost immunity and build resistance to infection. For instance, in a group of 100 elderly patients, low blood levels of vitamin E were associated with an increased number of infections.[7] In another study, vitamin E supplementation was shown to increase resistance to a number of infectious agents.[8] These are but two of many studies that have begun to verify the link between nutrition and immunity.

A case can also be made that even when antibiotics are used, it is important that nutrients be supplemented as well. In 1985, a report in *The Lancet* described a woman suffering from trichomonal vaginitis and low blood levels of zinc who responded to drug treatment *only* after supplements raised her zinc level to normal.[9] In Chapter 2, we discussed a report showing that vitamin C, when used along with tetracycline, was associated with a 3- to 15-fold rise in the blood level of the antibiotic.[10] This would appear to be beneficial (if an antibiotic is needed), since an elevated blood level of antibiotic would optimize its effectiveness, minimize the adverse intestinal effect (since more is absorbed) and probably reduce the duration of antibiotic treatment. Another study showed that a zinc-erythromycin solution worked better for acne than erythromycin alone.[11]

How Infection Affects Nutritional Status

Not only does nutritional deficiency affect resistance to infection. Infection itself can alter nutritional status. Doctors have known for many years, for example, that conditions such as rheumatoid arthritis, acute tonsillitis, fever, pneumonia, and measles result in inadequate amounts of vitamin A in the tissues. These conditions often lead to depletion of vitamin A, which renders one more susceptible subsequent infections.

In 1987, an article in the *American Journal of Clinical Nutrition* raised some very interesting points about nutrition and infection. Dr. F.A. Campos and his colleagues found that after an episode of chickenpox, children had inadequate body reserves of vitamin A for three months or longer after the infection.[12] Commenting on this and similar studies of measles, Dr. Thomas R. Frieden of the New York City Department of Health states, "In developing countries, children who survive measles have increased morbidity [illness] and mortality [death] from respiratory infections and diarrhea for at least 1 year. Since vitamin A deficiency increases the severity of bacterial, viral, and parasitic infections, and is associated with increased diarrheal morbidity and mortality, the decline in total body stores of vitamin A caused by measles may contribute to increased postmeasles mortality."[13]

Deficiency of nutrients prior to or as a result of infection has important consequences. As Dr. Frieden's groups showed, children with measles who had low levels of vitamin A, were more likely to have fever and to be hospitalized. Other studies have shown that such children are more likely to suffer from pneumonia and diarrhea.

Another group of nutrients adversely influenced by infection is the essential fatty acids. These fats play an important role in regulating inflammation and immune function. Infection by the Epstein-Barr virus, associated with some cases of chronic fatigue syndrome and immune dysfunction, blocks the body's ability to manufacture vital compounds known as prostaglandins. Other viruses are known to do the same. When this occurs, susceptibility to infection by bacteria or reinfection by viruses increases. In people who do not seem to recover from an infection, blood and tissue levels of certain fatty acids (e.g. GLA and EPA) are depressed when compared with those who recover from such infections.[14] When essential fatty acids are given as a supplement, resistance to infection improves markedly.

These studies suggest that infection can cause the loss of nutrients important to immune function. Unless corrected, these deficiencies can render a child or adult susceptible to future viral, bacterial or parasitic illness. This is not a new discovery. In 1976, researchers discovered that during infection, levels of vitamin C in the blood and tissues fell so low that the mechanisms used by white cells to attack bacteria was impaired. At such low levels, one is at risk to secondary infection. Similar findings have been reported with zinc and magnesium. Other nutrients are probably also effected.

One wonders why medical physicians continue to ignore the growing evidence that nutrition influences infection susceptibility and that infection further degrades nutritional status. Logic would suggest that all patients suffering from infection would at least receive some form of nutritional support. But this is not the standard of care in the U.S. Other providers such as chiropractors, naturopaths and holistic M.D.s must take the lead in this regard. It seems negligent on the part of doctors to ignore such basic factors that influence health!

Food Allergy, Intolerance and Immunity

Allergy or intolerance to foods is one of the most commonly over-looked contributors to altered immunity and susceptibility to infection. According to James C. Breneman, M.D., former chairman of the Food Allergy Committee of the American College of Allergists, "The incidence of food allergy is greater than the incidence of any other type of illness affecting mankind. By some estimates, 60 percent of the population has unknown food intolerances or allergies. This constitutes a hidden iceberg of food allergy with only a small percentage, roughly 5 percent, of the iceberg showing. The other 95 percent of the food allergy patients go about their suffering unrecognized and untreated."

If food allergy and intolerance are so prevalent, why do most doctors seem to ignore their existence? Dr. Breneman shares his view on this when he states, "A society has developed that suffers increasingly from food allergy and intolerance while inadequate numbers of professional people have been educated to cope with the problem. Medical school curricula usually offer studies in allergy as elective courses. The student is taught allergy, not as a primary science, but as an art subordinate to the Department of Internal Medicine or Pediatrics."[15]

Dr. Breneman uses the terms "allergy" and "intolerance" when describing adverse reactions to food. This is an important distinction. True allergy involves a response by the immune system. Allergists usually consider an adverse food reaction to be allergy only when elevated blood levels of certain antibodies, usually IgE (also IgG and IgM), are demonstrated. An example is the runny nose, sneezing and itchy eyes associated with hay fever. The term intolerance is used when there is an adverse food reaction due to almost any other cause. Many doctors note that this type of reaction is growing in frequency as we consume more processed food, are exposed to more synthetic chemicals and use more antibiotics.

There is an old adage that says, "Allergy doesn't cause everything, but it can cause anything." Research and clinical experience have shown this to be true. Food intolerance has been associated with many disorders typically thought due to infection by bacteria. A classic example is ear infection in children. At the 1991 meeting of the American College of Allergy and Immunology, Dr. T. M. Nsouli presented a study of 104 children with chronic middle ear "infections." Seventy-eight percent of these children tested positive for reactivity to foods. After excluding offending foods from the diet for 11 weeks, 70 of 81 children experienced significant improvement. When offending foods were later reintroduced—to verify the significance of the food allergy—66 of the 81 children experienced aggravation of their middle ear condition.[16]

Tonsillitis has also been linked to food intolerance. According to an article published in the *Journal of the Royal Society of Medicine,* intolerance to cow's milk may be one of the principal causes of chronic tonsillitis. Chronic tonsillitis frequently leads to overuse of antibiotics and eventual tonsillectomy. How many doctors have ignored the very simple measure of suggesting that their patients eliminate dairy products from the diet? What is to be lost by withholding antibiotics for a time while dairy products are removed?

Respiratory tract infections are often related to food or airborne allergy. According to William G. Crook, M.D., writing in *Pediatric Clinics of North America,* "I agree . . . that allergy of the respiratory tract almost always masquerades as respiratory tract 'infection.'" He also stressed the importance of cow's milk allergy as a causative factor in recurrent bouts of respiratory disease, including bronchitis and pneumonia.[17]

Bladder infections have been linked to food intolerance as have sinus infections. Dr. Schmidt reported on a child with impetigo, a staph infection of the skin, that only improved after wheat and other gluten-containing foods were removed from the child's diet.

The Most Common Offenders

Although almost any food can contribute to or cause sluggish immunity or susceptibility to infection, certain common offenders are the most likely culprits. If a mother is breastfeeding and her child suffers from chronic infections that may be linked to food, the most likely offenders in the mother's diet are cow's milk, peanuts and eggs. In an infant or toddler, cow's milk, peanuts, egg and soy account for roughly 80 percent of adverse reactions to food. In adults, the following foods are most commonly found to cause problems (though they also commonly cause problems in children):

- Dairy products, including milk, butter, cheese, yogurt, cottage cheese and ice cream.
- Wheat, including not only bread and cereal, but anything that contains wheat such as gravies, crackers and cookies.
- Eggs or anything containing eggs.
- Chocolate.
- Citrus, especially oranges and orange juice.
- Corn, or anything containing corn, such as corn flakes.
- Soy.
- Peanuts and other nuts.
- Shellfish.
- Sugar.
- Yeast.

The Trouble with Cow's Milk

Cow's milk is often touted on television as the "perfect food." It is supposedly needed by everyone. "If you don't drink milk, your bones will become brittle from osteoporosis" hint many advertisers and even some physicians. Yet, cow's milk consumption may contribute to many of the health problems commonly encountered in our society. Excessive consumption of cow's milk may be one of the major factors contributing to susceptibility to common infections.

According to Dr. Schmidt in his book *Childhood Ear Infections*, simply eliminating dairy products is often all that's required to solve the riddle of recurrent ear problems in children. These sentiments are echoed by Dr. Fred Pullen, an ear, nose and throat specialist in Miami, Florida. Patients are referred to Dr. Pullen for the sole purpose of having tubes surgically implanted in their eardrums. Before undergoing surgery, however, all patients are first placed on a diet that eliminates dairy products. The result: "three-fourths [of these children] never need tubes."[18] The problems with cow's milk are so numerous that noted professor of pediatrics at Johns Hopkins School of Medicine, Dr. Frank Oski, wrote a book entitled *Please, Don't Drink Your Milk.*

What Causes Food Allergy and Intolerance?

Food allergy and intolerance are caused or aggravated by many, many factors. Some people have a genetic predisposition to the development of allergy. Overuse of antibiotics may contribute to thinning of the intestinal lining, overgrowth of yeast, susceptibility to invasion by parasites, poor absorption of nutrients and ultimately the development of intolerance to food. Overuse of antacids or anti-inflammatory drugs such as aspirin or ibuprofen also may lead to the development of intestinal "leakage" and development of food intolerance.

Infection of the intestines by viruses, bacteria or parasites also contributes to food intolerance. In one study of patients infected with the common parasite *Giardia lamblia,* 100 percent were intolerant of the milk sugar lactose. Doctors have known for years that viral infection of the intestine results in temporary intolerance to food. For example, children who experience diarrhea due to the common rotavirus suffer from food intolerance that lasts several weeks. If antibiotics are used in such infections, the likelihood of encouraging the development of allergy to food increases.

When the number of acidophilus and bifidus bacteria become too low (due to antibiotic use or for other reasons), the tendency to develop intolerance to food increases. Consumption of heavily chlorinated tap water is another means by which these bacteria are reduced.

Poor nutritional habits also contribute to development of food intolerance. Consumption of the wrong types of fats, too much sugar, too much junk food, too little fiber, too few vegetables and too little fruit makes it difficult for the absorption of nutrients to take place properly. It also makes it difficult to build new cells that line the digestive tract.

Testing if You're Allergic

You can discover whether your problems may be related to food allergy or intolerance by looking in three areas: history, symptoms and allergy tests.

History

- Do you have a family history of allergy?
- Did (or do) your mother, father or siblings suffer from allergy?
- Did you suffer from allergies as a child?

A history of allergy strongly suggests that allergy or intolerance may be hiding beneath your present problems.

Symptoms

Do you experience any of the common symptoms typically associated with allergy or intolerance to food? These fall into four basic areas:

1. respiratory symptoms such as coughing, wheezing, sinus or nasal congestion, bronchial congestion, frequent colds or earaches.
2. intestinal symptoms such as bloating, cramps, diarrhea, constipation, nausea, gas, loss of appetite or vomiting.
3. skin symptoms such as hives, eczema or non-specific rashes.
4. irritability, tension, fatigue, headache, insomnia or depression.

If you have one or more of these symptoms it may suggest allergy or intolerance to food. There are also physical signs such as puffy eyes, bags under the eyes, wrinkles under the eyes or patches of dry skin on the face or body that may signal allergy or intolerance to food.

Testing

The third important aspect in identifying whether food allergy or intolerance exists is the actual testing. This can be done in three basic ways: blood tests, skin tests or food-elimination tests.

Allergists commonly perform scratch tests of the skin, but this is not always accurate in identifying allergy or intolerance to food. According to allergist Albert Rowe, M.D., "It is generally agreed that clinical allergy may exist in the absence of positive skin reactions, especially those to the scratch test. This is true primarily in food allergy and to a lesser extent in inhalant allergy."[19] Another skin test in common use is the intradermal cutaneous test, in which a small amount of a suspected offender is injected just beneath the surface of the skin. The doctor observes the area for a characteristic reaction.

Blood tests in use today include serum tests for antibodies designated IgE, IgG and IgM. These tests look for proteins produced by the immune system in response to offending substances. Another test called the Leukocyte Histamine Release test (MetaMetrix Medical Research Laboratory, Norcross, GA) is also helpful in identifying the presence of allergy. In this test, an allergen is incubated in blood while the technician tests for the presence of histamine. Release of histamine indicates reactivity to the test substance.

The ELISA/ACT test (Serammune Physician's Lab, Reston, VA) is a well-researched tool for assessing allergic sensitivity. It measures primarily the delayed-type, or late-phase, allergic reactions. These are the ones most commonly missed with traditional allergy tests. ELISA/ACT measures reactivity to environmental chemicals, foods, environmental allergens (molds, dust, mites), airborne allergens (pollen), food additives, and preservatives. It is among the most comprehensive tools for assessing one's sensitivity to the environment and to food.

One of the most widely accepted forms of testing is the elimination-provocation test. To use this method, one is first placed on a diet that excludes foods that commonly trigger allergic reactions. The diet is continued for one to four weeks. After this time, suspected foods are added back to the diet one at a time. If any food produces symptoms upon reintroduction, the food is deemed an offender and must be avoided. Elimination-provocation is still considered the "gold standard" among allergy tests. Its main limitation is that it requires time, effort and compliance on the part of the patient.

Nutritional Deficiency: More Common Than You Think

Despite the abundance of food in the United States, nutritional deficiency is quite common. It is important to understand this because Americans are often lulled into believing that foods are fortified with needed nutrients, and besides, "the government is looking out for our health." We will need to first accept the fact that nutrient deficiency is common and then act to change the situation.

Pregnant women in the United States are frequently deficient in vitamins and minerals. In one study, 78 percent were seriously deficient in one or more nutrients.[20] In one analysis of elderly people, zinc intake was below the RDA in more than 90 percent.[21] Children and teenagers are especially susceptible to zinc deficiency because of their increased requirements for growth and development.[22] In a study of U.S. women, 20 to 40 percent had vitamin C intakes well below the very conservative RDA.[23]

Many children are deficient in nutrients vital to immune function. Leo Galland, M.D., author of *SuperImmunity for Kids,* sums it up this way: "Unfortunately, American children today get most of their calories from sugar, processed cereal grains such as wheat and corn, processed oils, dairy products, and fatty meats. It's no wonder that most children today consume less than two-thirds of the Recommended Dietary Allowance (RDA) of magnesium, vitamin B_6 and copper."

"Zinc and vitamin A deficiencies are very common, too. A zinc deficiency is most likely to occur in the young child who gets most of her nutrition from milk and cheese. Vitamin A deficiencies most often show up in adolescents who live on meat, potatoes, and fast foods, and who shun vegetables and eggs."[24]

According to work compiled by Melvyn R. Werbach, Clinical Professor at UCLA School of Medicine, many Americans do not meet the RDA for numerous vitamins and minerals, including: niacin, riboflavin, pyridoxine, pantothenic acid, thiamine, vitamin C, vitamin E, vitamin A, calcium, magnesium, zinc, selenium and more.[25]

Food, Nutrition and Infection Susceptibility

It comes as little surprise that the nutritional status of Americans has declined to this degree. Dr. Joseph Beasley summarizes USDA figures that reflect the changing dietary habits responsible for this:[26]

Soft drink consumption rose 182 percent from 1960–1981.

Food color consumption rose 1,006 percent from 1940–1981.

Corn syrup consumption rose 291 percent from 1960–1981.

From 1910 to 1976 fresh produce consumption *dropped* sharply.

Fresh apples................... down 75 percent

Fresh cabbage .... down 65 percent

Fresh fruit.................... down 33 percent

Fresh potatoes................ down 74 percent

Fresh melons .... down 50 percent

Soft drink consumption has actually outpaced consumption of *water* in the United States. Luc DeSchepper, M.D., Ph.D., author of *Peak Immunity,* reports that in 1986, Americans drank 42 gallons of soft drinks per capita, while consuming only 41 gallons of water. In 1964 the per capita consumption of water was 72 gallons compared with only 17 gallons of soft drinks. This change is one contributor to our declining levels of health. In one survey, almost 50 percent of children three to eight years of age drank soft drinks, as did 40 percent of children aged one to two.[27] The average soft drink contains roughly nine teaspoons of sugar! Far too much for anyone. In addition, the phosphoric acid present in many cola soft drinks causes the rapid elimination of magnesium in the urine.

We (the authors) recently conducted an informal survey of the common selections available on children's menus at various popular restaurants in the Minneapolis area. We were somewhat surprised to find unusual consistency. Whether the restaurant was Italian, Chinese, Dutch, Thai or American, the following items typically appeared:

- Cheeseburger, french fries and soft drink.
- Chicken nuggets, french fries and soft drink.
- Grilled cheese sandwich, french fries and soft drink.
- Hot dog, french fries and soft drink.

These foods are far too high in salt, fat, trans fatty acids and sugar.

What Affects Your Nutritional Needs

Individual nutritional needs vary tremendously, based on a number of factors. Genetic differences may cause basic needs to be different. Infection causes the need for certain nutrients to increase. Trauma or injury causes the need for nutrients used for tissue repair to go up. Alcohol consumption, especially if heavy, causes loss and destruction of most of the B-vitamins and many others. Stress increases the need for certain nutrients. During pregnancy, the need for folic acid, iron, zinc, essential fatty acids, calcium, magnesium and many other nutrients goes up substantially. During periods of rapid childhood growth, zinc, iron, calcium, protein and other nutrients must be present in greater amounts. As one ages, nutritional needs change as well.

People who are overweight or obese also have special nutritional needs. Obesity, paradoxically, is a condition of malnutrition. Consumption of excess calories often leads to excessive weight, but the calories are commonly empty so nutrient deficiency ensues. One often thinks of nutritional *deficiency* as a contributor to infection susceptibility. However, *excessive* intake of food and calories, as is common in Western societies where food is plenty, can lower immunity as well. This was shown years ago when dogs fed high-calorie diets, to the point of obesity, became much more susceptible to infection with canine distemper. Those with the highest caloric intake were also more likely to suffer paralysis from distemper than their infected counterparts on lower-calorie diets.[28]

Taking the concept further, Jeffrey Bland, Ph.D., nutritional biochemist and leading lecturer in the field of nutritional medicine, coined the phrase "overconsumptive undernutrition" many years ago. He referred to overconsumptive undernutrition as a state in which caloric intake is high, but nutrient density is low. The food contains plenty of calories, but many of the nutrients have been stripped through food processing. All of these calories must be metabolized by the body, yet there are insufficient vitamins and minerals available to do this. Body reserves must then be utilized, which leads to a gradual depletion of stored nutrients. This can result in deficiency of important nutrients.

Unfortunately, efforts to lose weight often cause muscle to be lost, resulting in further nutritional problems. It is not uncommon for an individual to go on a weight loss program and develop tonsillitis, sinusitis, a cold, the flu or another "opportunistic infection." This is because many weight loss programs contribute to protein starvation. During protein starvation, immune function decreases. That is why muscle is lost rather than fat. The body is trying to compensate for inadequate dietary protein by using its reserves—the muscles.

Dr. Bland, director of HealthComm in Gig Harbor, Washington, has developed weight loss programs and formulations that encourage weight loss from *fat,* not muscle. When compared with most of the popular weight loss programs, Dr. Bland's has proven superior in this regard. An added benefit of Dr. Bland's Ultra-Clear® is that it aids in detoxification of the body, meaning it encourages the elimination of environmental toxins that build up in the body over time.

Our nutritional needs are variable and they change over time. This is why the ultimate health promotion strategy is one tailored to meet each individual's body chemistry and circumstances.

Excess Sugar and Fat Can Lower Immunity

In 1951, Benjamin Sandler, M.D., a physician from North Carolina, wrote a book entitled *Diet Prevents Polio.* Dr. Sandler's work with rabbits and monkeys convinced him that high amounts of sugar in the diet made one more susceptible to polio. During the polio epidemic of 1948–49, he appeared on an Asheville radio station urging parents not to feed their children refined sugar or foods containing sugar such as ice cream, candy, and soft drinks. His admonitions also ran in local newspapers. In 1948, the incidence of polio in North Carolina was 2,402 cases. In 1949, after adopting the "Sandler diet," the rate had fallen to 214 cases. During this time, the national incidence of polio (39 states) had risen.[29] Was it a coincidence that the rate of polio dropped as the rate of sugar consumption decreased in this state? Did removal of sugar from the diet improve resistance to polio? It is difficult to *prove*, but there is good reason to believe that sugar consumption lowers immunity. In a report published in the *American Journal of Clinical Nutrition*, 100 grams of sugar from glucose, fructose, sucrose, honey or orange juice caused a *significant decrease* in the ability of white blood cells to engulf and destroy bacteria. This decrease in immune function was still present five hours after sugar was consumed.[30]

There are at least three other studies that show decreases in immune function following sugar consumption. It is probably not significant when one only consumes sugar on occasion. However, on a daily basis it can wreak havoc on your immune system. The problem is sugar creeps into virtually every aspect of our diet, often without our awareness. This is because sugar is added to almost every packaged food sold today. The average American consumes more than 130 pounds of sugar each year! This is 14 times more than was ingested only 100 years ago. It's far too much for our bodies to handle.

Breakfast cereal is another problem. Many of the most popular children's cereals contain almost 50 percent of their calories as sugar. The presence of large amounts of sugar in the diet causes a gradual depletion of zinc in the body. As zinc levels decline, the sense of taste declines as well. As taste perception declines, there is a greater need to flavor the food in order to make it "taste good." Usually this means putting more sugar on the cereal. This leads to a further reduction in body zinc levels, which further lowers the taste perception. As a result, a child heaps more sugar on top of his cereal. The cycle goes on and on.

In his book *Fighting the Food Giants*, biochemist Paul A. Stitt says that it is no accident that children's cereals are highly sugared. Food manufacturers were the first to discover that sugar consumption leads to a gradual loss of zinc, which in turn leads to a loss of taste perception.[31] By marketing cereal high in sugar, they were able to create virtual addicts to their products. What parent has not heard the screams of a toddler in the grocery store demanding his breakfast treat!

Kids enjoy sweet foods. They are unlikely to persist long on any diet that completely eliminates sweets. You must gradually add naturally sweetened foods such as fruit to the diet. There are many food items other than refined sugar that lend a sweet taste to any food. These include:

- Honey
- Pear juice
- Dates
- Raisins
- Rice syrup
- Sorghum
- Maple syrup

A person with allergies may be sensitive to some of the above, so be alert for changes in mood, behavior or health when you first introduce these foods. If you or your child are yeast-sensitive or suffer from intestinal yeast problems, avoid feeding additional sugars. In general, use *all* sweeteners sparingly—even those listed above.

Excessive fat in the diet has also been shown to lower immune function. It seems that when blood levels of fat are too high, the ability of white blood cells to gobble bacteria decreases significantly. If your cholesterol or triglycerides are above normal, it may be interfering with your ability to fight infection. Also, if dietary fat intake is too high, it would be wise to replace it with low-fat foods. If you go on a weight loss program, make sure it is one that does not encourage the loss of muscle. You may wish to contact Health-Comm, Inc. of Gig Harbor, Washington, for information on this topic.

The Importance of Fiber

Fiber, or roughage, has been a popular topic in the media of late. While advertisers try to sell us many things we don't need, they're right when they say high-fiber cereals are important for good health. Lack of fiber has been implicated in the development of colon disease, heart disease and numerous other conditions. Dr. Denis Burkitt was the first to advance the idea of fiber as an important contributor to health. He based his beliefs on his research of African tribes. Dr. Burkitt found that African tribal residents suffered from almost none of the modern diseases of the West such as colon cancer and heart disease. However, when the Africans moved to the West and adopted our eating habits, they quickly succumbed to our most common illnesses.

Dietary fiber is as important to kids as it is to adults. Foods high in fiber are high in vitamins, trace minerals and essential fatty acids. Take wheat for example. Almost all of the essential nutrients are bound in the germ portion of the grain. During milling, the germ is separated from the endosperm. The germ is sold separately as wheat germ (long known as a high-nutrient food) while the endosperm is further milled to make flour. Milling of whole grain to make refined flour results in loss of 85 percent of the magnesium, 86 percent of the manganese, 40 percent of the chromium, 78 percent of the zinc, 89 percent of the cobalt, 48 percent of the molybdenum and 68 percent of the copper, in addition to comparable losses of selenium, vitamin E and essential fatty acids.[32] Moreover, heavy metals such as cadmium (which are concentrated in the endosperm) remain in the flour. (Unfortunately, the body's antagonist to cadmium—zinc—has been removed.) Since nutrients are required to properly utilize all calories we consume, the intake of refined foods leads to a gradual deficiency of nutrients. This is a strong argument for the use of whole-grain products.

Think about a typical breakfast. If you consume white bread with butter and peanut butter along with Rice Crispies and milk, you are getting very little fiber. Moreover, you are getting none of the important essential fatty acids. Most of the fat in this meal is saturated fat. White bread and Rice Crispies are fortified with a few token nutrients, but it is nothing when compared with the nutrients removed in processing.

Compare this with a breakfast of whole wheat bread using walnut butter as a spread, a whole orange, cooked rolled-oat cereal and yogurt. This breakfast has more vitamin C, magnesium, selenium, essential fatty acids and fiber than the one above with only a fraction of the saturated fat. Those who follow a diet such as this are generally healthier than those who follow a diet like the all-too-common one above.

The real test of the value of refined (fortified) foods would be to put a group of lab animals on a diet of white bread and compare them to a group fed a diet of whole-grain bread. In one such experiment, two-thirds of rats kept on a diet of enriched white bread died before the experiment was finished.[33]

Fiber is also important because it helps keep the intestinal contents moving through to their ultimate fate—elimination as stool. If the intestinal contents move too slowly, toxic by-products of digestion and bacterial fermentation remain in the bowel too long and are reabsorbed back into the body. Over time, this can contribute to illness.

When one consumes a diet low in fiber, attachment of parasites such as *Giardia lamblia* is easier. When fiber is present in the diet, the intestinal contents move through more quickly and prevent the attachment of such parasites. Recall that *G. lamblia* is one of the most common parasites found in the United States. It contributes to immune suppression, poor digestion, food allergies and numerous other problems. The ability to decrease the likelihood of infection by this parasite by simply increasing the intake of fiber is significant.

While fiber is necessary for children and adults, too much fiber can be a problem as well, since excessive fiber can cause nutrients to be leached out of the digestive tract. The problems for most of us, however, is not too much fiber, but too little. (Never put a child on a *high*-fiber diet without consulting a health care professional.) Good sources of fiber include fruit, vegetables, legumes and grains (oats, wheat, rice, barley, etc.).

Anti-Nutrients and Immunity

Anti-nutrients are substances to which we are all exposed through food and water that antagonize nutrients needed for health. Some anti-nutrients bind to other nutrients, making them useless. Others tie up enzymes needed in digestion and other body functions. Some cause problems by creating a greater need for certain nutrients. Others cause nutrients to be excreted more rapidly from the body. In our world of high technology, the level of anti-nutrients to which we are exposed is surprisingly high. Many of the anti-nutrients have a direct or indirect effect on immune function. Anything you can do to reduce exposure to anti-nutrients will be helpful in preventing recurrent illness.

Sugar, food coloring, processed fats, additives like BHT, and most of the 3,000 or so food additives allowed in the United States often act as anti-nutrients. Pesticides used to grow food can remain on food and act as anti-nutrients. For example, in 1985 it was reported that American agriculture uses 1 billion pounds of pesticides each year. That is 4.5 pounds for every man, woman and child in the country.[34] These chemicals have many potential adverse effects. They will be discussed further in Chapter 5.

Prescription drugs constitute another important category of anti-nutrients. If drug therapy is short, the effects are usually not severe. However, if one takes a drug for months or years, the nutritional effects of the drugs *must* be taken into account. If you are on medication, it is important that you discuss this with your doctor. If your doctor prescribes medication but fails to address the nutrient effects of the medication, it may be wise to seek a doctor who will take this into account. Below is just a sample of the nutrients adversely affected by drugs.

Drug	Clinical Condition	Nutrient Affected
Antibiotics	bacterial infection	vit. K, A, B_{12}, Mg, folic acid, C, K+
Aspirin	pain, fever	B_1, vit. C, K+
Cortisone	inflammation, allergy	Zn, K+, folate, B_6, vit. C, D, Ca
Ritalin	hyperactivity, ADD	suppress appetite
Phenobarbital	seizure disorders	vit. C, D, Ca, Mg, folic acid
Tetracyclines	infection	Zn, Ca, Fe, Mg, vit. K B_2, B_3, C, folate

The Eating Environment

Little consideration is given today to the importance of the traditional sit down meal. Parents and children are running off in different directions to make PTA appointments, soccer practice, dance classes and cub scouts. Meals are sometimes consumed with a speed that would make even the most voracious canine blush. The relative calm that presided at mealtime in decades past no longer exists in most families. "So what?" you may say.

How you eat may not be as important as what you eat, but it does have an impact. As researchers begin to look at the importance of mind and emotions on immune function, it has become clear that digestive function is also affected. For instance, the output of digestive enzymes is dramatically affected by the activity one engages in while eating. Those who perform "left brain" tasks such as reading or mathematics have significantly lower output of digestive enzymes than do those who meditate or sit quietly during meals. (One can almost envision the harried accountant during tax season, a sandwich in one hand and an adding machine at the other.) There are indications that haste or stress during mealtime might have the same effect.

Why is this important? Nutrient availability is dependent upon the digestive system's ability to properly break down and absorb vitamins and minerals. If enzymes are not produced in adequate amounts, foods are not broken down properly, vitamins and minerals are not released, nutrients are not absorbed and the body gravitates toward a gradual state of deficiency. Enzymes also protect against viral, bacterial and parasitic infection of the digestive tract.

According to a survey commissioned by Ketchum Advertising of San Francisco, 62 percent of dinners eaten at home are spent with the TV on, breakfast takes an average of 18 minutes to eat, while dinner takes an average of 30 minutes.[35] This is not the optimum way to enhance digestion.

The solution is to make mealtime more sacred, more relaxed. It should be a time when everyone sits down together—peacefully. No radio, no television, no newspaper. No rushing around. The environment should be as serene as possible—even with a toddler or five-year-old.

Food, Nutrition and Coping

In Chapter 7, the effect of emotional stress on immunity is discussed. You will learn that our ability to cope with stressful circumstances has much to do with whether our immune systems become depressed during stress and whether we succumb to infections. Coping is generally considered a psychological response. However, there are dietary and nutritional factors that can have a profound effect on the ability of both children and adults to cope with stresses in their world. In some cases, the nutritional factors prevent us from being able to cope with even normal day-to-day events. This is not surprising when you realize that the brain has the highest concentration of nutrients of any organ in the body.

Consider the trace element magnesium. Magnesium deficiency has been associated with symptoms such as anxiety, confusion, hyperactivity, insomnia, irritability, nervousness and restlessness. Magnesium deficient individuals also are commonly hypersensitive to noise. The typical person with these characteristics often "flies off the handle" with minimal provocation. Trivial events seem threatening. The noise created by a cadre of children or grandchildren is enough to trigger outbursts of hostility or anger. If one tends to hold their feelings inside, the mounting pressure building within causes blood pressure to rise. Others are likely to lash out easily when stressful circumstances present. When supplemented with magnesium, such individuals often improve dramatically—their "coping" skills are enhanced.

Dr. Smith has studied the nutritional status of more than 8,000 hyperactive children. He notes that magnesium deficiency is a common finding in such children. Hyperactive children are notorious for their poor coping skills. They are nervous, anxious, inattentive, restless, impatient and startled by the slightest sound. They place extreme demands upon the patience of their parents. Dr. Smith remarks that hyperactive children are more likely to be abused by their parents because such children frequently push their parents beyond the limits of tolerance. When optimal nutritional status is maintained for these kids, their hyperactive behavior frequently improves, as does their ability to cope with stressful stimuli.

Food allergies also can have a dramatic effect on brain biochemistry, leading to changes in coping ability. They can turn a bright, witty, articulate person into a dull, depressed, irritable and sometimes confused human being. In his book *Brain Allergies*, William Philpott, M.D., describes two cases that illustrate this point:

1. "A twelve-year-old boy diagnosed as hyperkinetic had the following symptoms on testing for spinach: he became overtalkative and physically violent, had excessive saliva, was very hot, developed a severe stomach-ache, and cried for a long time. Watermelon made him irritable and depressed; cantaloupe made him aggressively tease other patients. Once he avoided the incriminating substances in his diet, his hyperkinesis symptoms diminished dramatically."

2. The case of a thirty-six-year-old woman: "Pineapple evoked irritability, blocking of thought, dizziness, and a severe headache. . . . Oranges made her violently angry, and she fought with her son; her mind functioned so poorly she could hardly carry on a conversation. Rice brought on uncontrollable giggling followed by crying."[36]

It takes no medical training to realize that neither of these individuals would be able to cope well with stressful stimuli. They exhibited a collapse in their coping skills with no provocation other than a change in food consumption.

Studies have also shown that some people with intestinal overgrowth of yeast convert dietary sugar into alcohol. The alcohol is then absorbed into the bloodstream. Blood levels of alcohol are increased even though the person has consumed no alcohol. In some cases, the blood alcohol is found at levels that would qualify the subjects as legally drunk. Might this not have a dramatic effect on coping ability? Might it not have an effect upon perception of events—stressful or otherwise?

Food and nutrition have a direct and profound effect upon our ability to tolerate stress. Poor dietary choices, nutrient-deficient foods, food high in synthetic additives, food allergies or individual biochemical imbalances affect brain chemistry and must be considered when calculating the toll of stress in our lives.

Thyroid Problems and Altered Immunity

One of the most commonly overlooked contributors to lowered immunity is hypothyroidism (low thyroid function). The thyroid gland is responsible for maintaining proper body temperature and for energy production within every cell. People who suffer from low thyroid function are frequently cold even when others in the room might be comfortable or perhaps even warm. When body temperature is low due to poor thyroid function the body's white blood cells behave sluggishly. When body temperature is high, as in fever, infection-fighting ability improves. An increase of two degrees centigrade of fever, for instance, has been shown to increase T-cells and antibodies by 2,000 percent over the numbers present at normal body temperature.

In his fascinating book about thyroid problems entitled *Solved: The Riddle of Illness,* Stephen E. Langer, M.D. discusses the link between thyroid function and immunity in some detail. In Chapter 4 he writes, "Subnormal body temperature and too little thyroid hormone can reduce the strength and resistance of every cell, including the billions involved in the immune system. One of the most common results of hypothyroidism which I see daily in my office is recurrent colds, throat and nose infections and other respiratory ailments."* Hypothyroidism can also contribute to depression and poor coping ability, both associated with lowered immunity.

The connection between hypothyroidism and infection susceptibility is especially significant if you consider the estimate by Broda Barnes, M.D., that possibly 40 percent of the American population is hypothyroid. Dr. Barnes is a specialist in endocrinology and has worked with thyroid disorder for several decades. He contends that blood tests are often not sensitive in detecting poor thyroid function because blood values change only after the condition has existed for some time. Based on the knowledge that low thyroid function lowers body temperature, Dr. Barnes devised a simple test that can be easily applied at home called the Basal Temperature Test. The test is done as follows: Shake down a thermometer and leave it on the nightstand before going to bed. When you awaken in the morning, remain in bed and place the thermometer snugly in your armpit for 10 minutes. It is important that you do not get out of bed before or during the test as physical

---

*Langer, SE, Scheer JF. *Solved: The Riddle of Illness,* New Canaan, Connecticut: Keats Publishing, 1984;38.

activity will elevate body temperature and give a false reading. Read the thermometer. The normal range for the axillary (underarm) temperature is 97.8 to 98.2. A lower temperature suggests hypothyroidism. The test should be conducted on three consecutive days. Women obtain the best results when not menstruating.

If your basal temperature is low, seek care from a doctor who will follow up with bloodwork. But remember, blood tests do not always detect thyroid problems that are marginal. Also, see Dr. Langer's book. If you seek care for low thyroid, realize that simply taking *synthetic* thyroid hormone is usually insufficient. The thyroid is highly dependent upon an adequate supply of nutrients including vitamins A, C, E, B_2, B_3, B_6, the trace elements zinc and copper, and essential fatty acids. Many doctors knowledgeable in nutritional medicine now prescribe these and other nutrients along with natural or desiccated thyroid tissue.

If you suffer form low immunity, feel as though you easily "catch" infectious illnesses, or suffer from chronic infections of the ear, nose, throat, lungs, skin, bladder, or vagina, a simple Basal Temperature Test may be the first step on your road to wellness.

Infections From Your Food

Most of our discussion thus far has focused on the role of diet and nutrition in immune function. However, there is another aspect of the food-infection connection that is gaining more attention. Intestinal infection by the food-borne bacteria such as *Salmonella* and *Campylobacter* is a growing problem in the United States. The most common source of this infection is poultry—chicken and eggs. According to a committee of the National Academy of Sciences, one in 50 people in the United States gets sick each year from *Salmonella* or *Campylobacter*. The almost 500,000 reported cases each year are considered only the tip of the iceberg. Some estimate that from 20 to 80 million people in the United States suffer from food poisoning each year.[37]

Food poisoning can occur following consumption of pork, beef, chicken, eggs, shellfish, sushi and dairy products. Symptoms include: nausea, abdominal cramps, diarrhea, fever, headache and sometimes vomiting.

Prevention

- Cook chicken and turkey thoroughly, until there are no pink juices running.
- Never let raw meat or its juices touch other food.
- Wash your hands and any utensils that have contacted raw meat in hot, soapy water.
- Don't use wooden cutting boards for meat. They harbor bacteria.
- Thaw frozen birds in the refrigerator, not in the microwave or on the counter.
- Keep your refrigerator below forty degrees Fahrenheit and your freezer at or below zero degrees.
- Buy free-range or organic animals. Avoid animals fed antibiotics.
- Avoid consuming raw egg yolk.

Home Care

If you experience diarrhea, abdominal cramps, fever or vomiting following a meal and suspect food poisoning, do the following:

- Take 1 teaspoon of acidophilus powder every hour until symptoms subside.
- Along with the acidophilus, take ½ teaspoon of Inner Strength® (see Chapter 10).
- Both can be mixed in warm water and taken together.
- If symptoms show no improvement in 24 to 48 hours, see your doctor.
- If you experience numbness, tingling or paralysis following a meal, seek emergency care immediately. This could be a sign of more serious food poisoning.

Eating For Optimum Immunity

It is beyond the scope of this book to present a detailed outline of an immune-boosting diet. However, eating healthy is a fairly simple process when certain concepts are understood. If you wish more specific information on immune building diets, consider the following books;

For general use: *Dr. Berger's Immune Power Diet.*

For those with chronic yeast-related illness: *The Yeast Connection Cookbook* by William G. Crook, M.D. and Marjory Hurt Jones, R.N.

For children: *SuperImmunity for Kids,* by Leo Galland, M.D. and Diane Dincin Buchman.

For those with environmental illness: *The Cure is in the Kitchen* by Sherry Rogers, M.D.

In general, we encourage our patients to avoid processed food. This is not always possible, but it is a worthy ideal.

Fiber: Consume fiber-containing foods every day. Sources include fruit, vegetables, legumes and grains.

Meat: Many of our modern-day illnesses stem from excessive consumption of meat, especially red meat. Red meat consumption should be restricted to two to three times a month. Fish and fowl are good sources of protein.

One need not become a strict vegetarian in order to be healthy. However, many people suffering from a variety of ills have found enormous relief and, in many cases, a cure after several months on a vegetarian diet.

If you are a strict vegetarian or are on a macrobiotic diet, you should have your vitamin B_{12} status checked, since many strict vegetarians are low in this vitamin. Children of vegetarian or macrobiotic mothers are also at risk for low vitamin B_{12}. In these tender years, deficiency of B_{12} can have serious neurologic implications. The solution is to consume some fish or take a B_{12} supplement. Nori and spirulina, two purported sources of B_{12} for vegetarians, have been shown to contain a form of B_{12} that is not utilized properly by the body.[38]

Sugar: Reduce your intake of sugar. Use natural sugars when necessary. Consume fruit.

Fat: Keep your intake of fat to about 20 percent of your total calories. The only exception is for infants and toddlers. Infants must get roughly 50 percent of their calories from fat. This gradually goes down as the child ages.

Eat more cold-water fish such as salmon, mackerel, herring,

sardines and trout. The fats and oils in these fish are very helpful and generally deficient in our Western diets. Also consume flax oil periodically. This contains omega-3 fatty acids commonly deficient in our diets.

Cook with olive oil and reduce your use of sunflower, safflower and corn oil. These latter oils are easily destroyed (or oxidized) when exposed to the high heat of cooking. If the temperature is kept low, these oils can be used sparingly. They can also be used raw. Buy cold-pressed oils when possible.

Avoid sources of trans fatty acids, or what have been dubbed "funny fats." Trans fatty acids created when unsaturated fats, such as that found in sunflower or safflower oil, are heated. Heating results in a change in the shape of the fat molecules, making them extremely harmful to the body. Deep-frying is one of the worst processes for bringing about such a change. Foods high in trans fats include chicken nuggets, french fries, pastries, corn chips, potato chips, candy, cakes, frosting, cookies, margarine, crackers and fish sticks. Avoid any food where the words "may contain the following" are followed by the words "partially hydrogenated." Up to 50 percent of the fat in these foods occurs as trans fatty acids. These can influence infection-fighting capability and inflammation and should be avoided.

Do You Need Vitamin and Mineral Supplements?

The question of whether the average person needs daily supplements is an area of some controversy. It is our opinion that nearly everyone can benefit from supplementation. This is especially true if one has a history of recurrent illness, eats poorly, is under stress, is on medication, has food or airborne allergies, or suffers from malabsorption or intestinal complaints. If supplementation is approached with reason and understanding, the chance for benefit is high, while the chance for harm is almost negligible.

The type and amount of supplements you take depend on your motives and individual circumstances. If you are healthy and want a prevention program, you would likely take smaller amounts than if you were ill and needed a therapeutic program. Vitamin C can be used to illustrate this point. A healthy person might do well on 500 mg per day, and do even better on 1,000 to 5,000 mg per day (or

1 to 5 grams). Should this person come down with tonsillitis or the flu, 20 to 30 grams might be more appropriate.

Another commonly asked question is whether megavitamin supplementation is helpful. In our opinion, there is a place for megavitamin supplements, but only if a health professional trained in clinical nutrition has determined that there is a specific need for large amounts of a certain nutrient. Whenever large amounts of one nutrient are given over time, there is a chance of creating deficiencies of other nutrients. Most people do not need megadoses. However, we also believe that the RDA has been set arbitrarily low for many important nutrients such as vitamin E, beta-carotene, vitamin C and others.

Immune-Boosting Nutrients

Scientists will probably some day discover that nearly all nutrients have some direct or indirect role in immune function. Some of the more thoroughly understood nutrients are being used in medicine to prevent infection and to boost immunity during infection. Those usually discussed include vitamin A, E, C, B-complex, beta-carotene, zinc, iron, selenium and coenzyme Q_{10}.

Vitamin A

Vitamin A is a powerful immune stimulant. It has been shown to increase the size of the master gland of the immune system, the thymus. When vitamin A levels are too low, the thymus shrinks, followed by a decrease in the number of circulating white cells. Vitamin A helps maintain the cells lining the lungs, intestinal tract and bladder. These cells are the first barrier of the protection mechanism against infection. When vitamin A is deficient, these cells begin to change, making the tissue susceptible to invasion by viruses, bacteria and parasites.

Vitamin A levels are depleted rapidly during different conditions, including fever, pneumonia, tonsillitis, rheumatic fever and measles. In one report of children with severe measles, the rate of complications such as pneumonia, croup and death was cut in half as a result of vitamin A supplementation.[39]

There is one caveat regarding vitamin A; it can be toxic at high doses (although there are annually only 200 reported cases of vitamin A excess worldwide).[40] More is not better. The RDA for children aged one to three is 2,000 units; for children aged four to five, 2,500 units. Children should not be given more than 10,000 IU/day unless prescribed by a doctor. Pregnant women and persons with liver disease, viral hepatitis or malnutrition should consult a doctor before taking vitamin A. When vitamin A is used to treat illness in adults, from 10,000 to 30,000 IU are often given. Vitamin A should not be consumed in large amounts for prolonged periods (more than 1–2 weeks) without consulting a doctor.

Beta-carotene

Beta-carotene is a fat-soluble nutrient found in orange, yellow and green vegetables such as carrots, squash and sweet potatoes. It is important as an antioxidant, meaning it protects cells against damage by free-radicals and damaging pollutant molecules. This nutrient is also important in immune function. Beta-carotene is a precursor to vitamin A, meaning that some beta-carotene is converted into vitamin A.

Vitamin E

Vitamin E exerts an effect on the immune system through its role as an antioxidant. This vitamin protects the fats and cell membranes in the body from oxidation or damage. When vitamin E levels are low, damage to cell membranes easily occurs. Vitamin E also affects immune function by regulating the formation of prostaglandins, the hormone-like substances derived from our dietary fats. Daily doses of vitamin E in the range of 50 to 100 IU are considered quite safe. There have been few problems associated with doses up to 800 IU. Beyond 1,200 IU, immune-suppressive effects have been reported. During illness, 400 to 800 IU is a reasonable dose. Any time supplementary foods containing essential fatty acids are consumed, such as flax oil, primrose oil or fish oil, additional vitamin E should be consumed.

Vitamin C

Vitamin C seems to influence resistance to bacterial and viral infections in two basic ways: by direct inhibition of the virus or bacteria and by stimulating white blood cells' ability to attack bacteria and viruses. One means by which white blood cells destroy bacteria is through a process called phagocytosis, meaning engulf and destroy. It was demonstrated almost fifty years ago that vitamin C is required for this process. When levels of ascorbic acid are too low, white blood cells are sluggish and inefficient in combating bacteria and viruses.

A typical scenario is as follows. A person consumes a diet only marginal in vitamin C. She is not deficient enough to show overt signs of scurvy, but her body is not functioning at its peak. Then a cold or flu strikes and rapidly depletes the remaining stores of vitamin C. Her immune system responds slowly, allowing the infection to gain a foothold. Depending on the severity of the vitamin C losses, susceptibility to secondary bacterial infections such as pneumonia may follow. Vitamin C also increases the rate at which white blood cells travel to the site of infection (called chemotaxis).[41]

It is known that dogs and other animals that make vitamin C increase production 10- to 15-fold during times of stress or infection. Since humans do not make vitamin C, it is necessary for us to get additional vitamin C from a supplement. It only makes sense that we increase our intake commensurate with our increased needs. See Chapter 8 for more details on vitamin C.

Zinc

Zinc is probably the most extensively studied nutrient relative to its role in infection and immunity. Zinc is relatively safe. However, it should not be consumed in amounts greater than 25 mg per day in healthy individuals. Individuals with skin problems, recurring infections, loss of taste sensation, etc., may need higher amounts until symptoms improve. Never take more than 75 mg per day unless directed by your doctor. In one study of 11 men who took 150 mg of zinc twice daily for 6 weeks, there was a reduction in immune function.[42] When doctors prescribe large doses of zinc, they generally monitor copper status and/or give a copper supplement concurrently with zinc.

The RDA for zinc in children is 10 mg per day and for adults, 25 mg per day. In a recent case of a child with acute glandular swelling of the neck, we used 75 mg of zinc plus 10,000 mg vitamin C for one week. This produced a rapid improvement in symptoms and since the dose was discontinued after one week, no risk of toxicity. We should mention that the boy's pediatrician wanted to prescribe an antibiotic, but the parents wanted to give nutritional therapy a chance. It worked.

Iron

Iron is essential for proper immune function. Susceptibility to infections is one of the common conditions associated with iron deficiency. Although iron deficiency can occur at any age, it is most common in children under age two (especially if bottlefed or consuming cow's milk), adolescent girls, some athletes and pregnant women.

Generally, iron should not be supplemented on a daily basis (except in bottlefed babies between six and twelve months), unless it has been established that iron deficiency exists. This can be determined by a blood test called a serum ferritin test. Hemoglobin is a useful screening test, but it is not always indicative of iron deficiency.

Selenium

Deficiency of selenium results in diminished resistance to bacterial and viral infections, diminished white blood cell activity, reduced antibody production and reduced ability of T-cells and natural killer cells to destroy pathogenic bacteria. Supplementation with selenium has been shown to reverse these processes. In one study, supplementation with selenium reduced the frequency of upper respiratory infections in children with Down syndrome.[43]

Selenium works with glutathione to act as one of the most potent antioxidant systems in the body. In this way, it protects the body from damage by chemicals in the environment. Selenium is usually taken in microgram amounts. Ten to 20 mcg per day is a common prevention amount. When doctors prescribe selenium, they will often use 100 to 800 mcg or more.

Coenzyme Q$_{10}$

This is a recent addition to our knowledge of the immune-building arsenal. CoQ$_{10}$ is a powerful antioxidant and immune stimulant.

Like vitamin C, vitamin E, beta-carotene and selenium, it is protective against free-radical damage that can occur with infection, aging and exposure to toxic chemicals. It is also important for generating energy within cells. Many people who suffer from chronic fatigue can benefit from Coenzyme Q_{10} supplementation. People who are immune-suppressed are commonly found to have low blood levels of this nutrient. Moreover, during infection, levels of CoQ_{10} decrease, leading to deficiency. Animals and humans who have been supplemented with this nutrient have been shown to have more active immune systems. People suffering from post-viral chronic fatigue syndrome often benefit enormously from CoQ_{10}. According to reports submitted to the FDA, this nutrient is non-toxic.

Regarding CoQ_{10} and immunity, Emile G. Bliznakov, M.D., Scientific Director of the Lupus Research Institute, asserts, "Overall, the action of CoQ_{10} on the immune system is profound; it promotes bioenergetic processes in the human immune cells that may prove to be the key to curing many of the diseases that ail us."[44]

In a prevention program, 5 to 10 mg of CoQ_{10} are usually recommended. During illness, 70 to 100 mg are often used. Under the supervision of a doctor, even greater amounts are administered. CoQ_{10} is found in high amounts in broccoli, spinach, sardines, mackerel, beef and eggs.

Thymus tissue

The thymus is considered the master gland of the immune system. Scientists have been studying ways to stimulate this gland for decades. They have learned that one way to enhance the function of this gland is to feed thymus tissue extract (derived from cattle) to people with suppressed immune systems. The extracts contain active substances that stimulate the activity of the thymus gland and improve resistance to infection. Only thymus tissue that has been defatted or azeotrophically processed should be used.

A good immune-building formula for adults might contain the following:

Vitamin A . . . . 2,000 IU

Vitamin E. . . . . 400 IU

Vitamin C	500 mg
Beta-carotene	100 mg
Vitamin B6	20 mg
Vitamin B5	30 mg
Zinc	10 mg
Copper	200 mcg
Selenium	50 mcg
CoQ10	10 mg
Bioflavonoids	150 mg

Vitamin C levels could ideally be increased to 1,000 to 6,000 milligrams per day during periods of wellness.

During periods of illness, all of the above can be increased substantially. However, vitamin A should not be increased beyond 25,000 IU per day for more than two or three weeks unless a doctor monitors your liver function. People with liver disease should not take this amount of vitamin A without first consulting a doctor. Zinc should not be taken in amounts greater than 75 mg per day for more than two weeks unless copper levels are monitored.

While nutritional supplements can often be used to overcome the ill health brought about by poor dietary habits, supplements *are never* a substitute for healthy eating habits. When one eats healthfully *and* takes supplements, the road to good health is made easier.

Nutrition has a profound effect on our resistance to disease. One is tempted to think that many or all infections can be prevented or treated with nutrition. Nutrition is always an important player in the game of building immunity, but it is not the only player. You will see that stress, lifestyle and environmental factors can overcome our limits even during conditions of optimum nutrition. Thus, we have to recognize nutrition's role and give it its rightful place on the wellness team.

A Summary of Things to Do

1. Reduce your intake of refined sugar. Excess sugar can make the immune system sluggish.

2. Reduce your intake of fat (unless it is already at or below 20 percent of your total calories). Avoid margarine and hydrogenated fats. If your triglycerides are high, work to lower them. Elevated blood fats can slow immune function.

3. Increase your intake of omega-3 essential fatty acids such as those found in flax oil and fish oil (salmon, mackerel, herring, sardines, trout). You may also wish to take a perle of evening primrose oil daily, which contains the omega-6 oil gamma-linolenic acid (GLA). Those in the industrialized world often consume too little of these oils. When taking additional oils *always* take additional vitamin E (50–400 mg).

4. Avoid white bread and refined flour products. They are devoid of essential nutrients including the essential fatty acids mentioned above.

5. Include fiber in your diet in the form of fruits, vegetables, nuts, seeds, legumes and whole grains. These foods are also high in vitamins and minerals.

6. Reduce your intake of pastries, doughnuts, french fries, chicken nuggets, candies and other foods containing "funny fats," or trans fatty acids. When these foods are consumed in excess, sluggish immunity may follow.

7. Eat several smaller meals a day as opposed to three large meals a day. It is easier on all aspects of your body.

8. Reduce your intake of coffee. Try the many varieties of herbal tea available.

9. Reduce your intake of soft drinks. They can leach calcium and magnesium from the body.

10. Follow the rhythms of your body. Eat when you're hungry, stop when you're full. Don't let the clock rule mealtime. Try mealtime without the paper, TV or radio.

11. Rotate your foods to avoid boredom and monotony. Eating the same foods every day can also lead to the development of food intolerance.

12. If you have a health problem, consider the possibility that the foods you consume might be part of the problem. Remember, allergies don't cause everything, but they can cause anything!

13. Take a multivitamin each day with meals. It should contain no artificial colors or preservatives and should be free of wheat, corn, soy, dairy and other products likely to cause problems in sensitive people.

14. Take extra vitamin C each day. 1,000 to 2,000 milligrams is a good start. Some believe higher amounts are even better.

15. Take other antioxidants such as beta-carotene, vitamin E and selenium. Antioxidants are important in immune function.

16. Don't be obsessive about nutrition. While a healthy, balanced diet is important to wellbeing, fretting about it may negate much of the good you've accomplished.

17. Splurge on your favorite treats now and then. If you've followed the guidelines above, reward yourself. Rigidity and abstinence are not the order of the day—just moderation and balance.

5

Environmental Threats to a Healthy Immune System

"Although the body's immune mechanisms have evolved over millions of years into an effective defense system, they can still be eluded—or damaged—by environmental agents."

Drs. R.S. Speirs and D.W. Roberts[1]

The spread of industrialization and technology development in the twentieth century knows no parallel in history. We have seen the emergence of some of the most dramatic and brilliant innovations ever conceived by humans. As our civilization embarked upon this journey of "progress," little thought was given to the consequences of such unbridled growth. With development has come growing environmental degradation. Our planet is now permeated with pollutants never dreamed of by our ancestors. The chemicals produced by industry and agriculture have now reached every corner of the globe. Indeed, there is not a place on the planet where DDT has not been found, even though its use was banned years ago. Other chemicals still in use contaminate the globe with greater frequency.

What this means is that no one is free from exposure to pollutants, however small. Exposure may come from fungicides on the food we eat, carbon monoxide drawn into our offices from city streets, formaldehyde used in construction of our homes, or benzene leached into our drinking water. With this has come a variety of diseases peculiar to the twentieth century, not to mention the rise of infections that were once controlled by proper hygiene and good nutrition.

In this chapter we look at some of the fundamental issues surrounding environment and its impact on immune function. We proceed from the assumption that everyone is exposed to one extent or another. Similarly exposed persons may react in entirely different ways. One may show no ill effects of low-level exposure. Another may react because of genetic differences. Yet another may suffer illness because poor nutrition has rendered him more susceptible to damage by toxic substances. In many instances, previously healthy people have been rendered immune-incompetent because of exposure to low levels of chemicals. Phil is a classic example.

Phil was a stockbroker and senior vice president of a large international brokerage company. A former runner, squash and tennis player and excellent physical specimen, Phil became debilitated after moving into a home that was later found to have been treated for termites. Phil could no longer run or play squash without severe pain and fatigue. He developed recurrent sinus infections and lower respiratory tract infections that were unresponsive to antibiotics. Phil's symptoms of environmental illness became so severe that he could no longer tolerate anything that was made or treated with synthetic chemicals. A wealthy man, Phil was resigned to buying old pieces of furniture at garage sales because they were made without chemicals. He drove an aging station wagon for the same reason.

After three years of nearly continuous antibiotic therapy for his recurrent infections, Phil sought the care of a physician practicing environmental medicine. Using diet, nutrition, homeopathic medicine and a detoxification program, Phil's sinus infections gradually came under control. There were dramatic changes in just one year. However, it took almost eight years to fully recover!

Robin was a chemist for a large Midwest manufacturing company. He was a healthy and active man with few health complaints. One day he advised his laboratory assistant to mix two chemicals together in preparation for an experiment. As the chemicals were being mixed, Robin realized he had given his colleague the wrong instruction. The chemical reaction caused a large cloud of vapor to permeate the lab. Robin was exposed briefly and from that day began to experience multiple health problems including recurrent sore throats, respiratory infections, chronic fatigue, headaches, dizziness, depression, food allergies and extreme sensitivity to perfumes and other environmental substances.

Robin saw some of the top physicians in occupational medicine in the Minneapolis area. All they could tell him was that he showed high levels of chemical by-products in his tissues and his immune system was not working. Robin then sought the care of a physician practicing environmental medicine. After numerous blood and urine tests that looked at Robin's metabolism, it became clear why many systems were not working—his immune system required significant minerals, vitamins and nutritional cofactors. After following a specially designed nutritional and detoxification program, Robin's health improved markedly.

Environmental Illness

Robin and Phil are examples of healthy people who developed chronic illness following exposure to some of our twentieth-century creations. They both developed what is now called environmental illness, or EI (sometimes called ESI, or environmental sensitivity illness). People with environmental illness are often said to be "allergic to the twentieth century." They suffer from chronic illness that is brought about by exposure to chemicals in their environment.

The symptoms have become so broad and seem to involve so many body systems that much of the medical profession has declared EI a "psychiatric illness." This is of little comfort to a person who is walking around with elevated blood levels of toluene metabolites or who develops pneumonia after breathing a cloud of automobile exhaust. The illness is real and the medical system is only beginning to recognize the true magnitude of the problem.

Toxins Inside and Out

The dictionary defines "toxic" as harmful or destructive. Something becomes toxic when it is present in amounts that exceed our ability to eliminate them without harm. For example, aspirin in small amounts can help relieve pain and reduce fever. In slightly greater amounts, aspirin can cause bleeding of the intestinal tract. In still greater amounts, aspirin can kill. Alcohol consumed in very small amounts has shown some benefit in cardiovascular health, yet in large amounts causes liver disease and death. So the question of toxicity is really one of degree.

Many substances only become toxic when they are present in certain amounts. Some substances are inherently more toxic than others. Death can result when only one drop of the toxin that causes botulism is ingested. Yet, it may take a quart of vodka to produce death.

Another factor comes into play. When certain toxins exist in low amounts in the presence of other toxins, their actions can be accentuated. For example, both aspirin and the food coloring yellow #5 can be toxic at certain levels. However, when present together they act in a synergistic way to produce sometimes-severe reactions. This can happen when one is exposed to only small amounts of each substance. In our modern world with tens of thousands of man-made chemicals circulating through the food, water and air, this type of synergistic effect is common.

There are both internal (or endogenous) and external (or exogenous) toxins that can affect our health. An internal toxin is something that is produced as a part of our normal bodily operations. An example is lactic acid. Lactic acid normally builds up in the muscles during prolonged exercise. Though not serious, lactic acid can produce a substantial amount of pain or stiffness in the muscles. Internal toxins can also be produced when normal operations go awry. External toxins are the most obvious to us. These are substances that we inhale through the air and ingest through food and drink. Lead, mercury, DDT and gasoline vapors are examples of external toxins.

Your Total Toxic Load

The way we are exposed to toxins from our internal and external environments can have an important effect on our health and immunity. Exposure to one large dose of the insecticide heptachlor can have serious lasting consequences on one's nervous and immune systems. Likewise, small amounts of a variety of toxic substances over time can have an additive effect on our bodies. Exposure to low amounts of formaldehyde in the home, gasoline from the garage, nitrogen oxides from the smog downtown, lead in the drinking water, colorings in the food, prescription drugs, etc., add up to what's known as the total toxic load. Individually, these substances may be present in such small amounts as to be insignificant. Collectively they add up to a heavy burden.

Much of the current toxicology research has involved studying the cancer-causing effects of different compounds tested individually. However, this is rarely the way in which we are exposed. Most of our exposure occurs in trace amounts from a wide array of substances slowly over time. If exposure to low levels of too many substances occurs for too long, it may eventually exceed the body's threshold of tolerance. The result—chronic illness.

Toxins from Within

Toxins can also be produced from bacteria, yeast and fungi that live in the intestines. These toxins are reabsorbed back into the bloodstream and must be processed or, if that is impossible, stored by the liver. In effect, a toxic waste dump develops. One obvious example of such a toxin is alcohol.

People who have chronic symptoms and suffer from chronic infections often have "dysbiosis" of the intestines, meaning an imbalance in the normal inhabitants of the gut. Overgrowth of yeast in the gut, usually *Candida albicans,* is part of the dysbiosis syndrome. When sugars are eaten, they eventually reach the colon where the yeast reside. It is a well-known fact that yeast ferment sugar into alcohol. This is how beer and wine are made (by mixing grain or grape juice with brewer's yeast). The bowel is no different. When yeast in the bowel begin to digest dietary sugars, they ferment them into alcohol. This is then absorbed into the blood. In some cases, this raises the blood alcohol to levels at which the person is considered legally drunk. This is the so-called "auto-brewery syndrome" or the "still in the gut" and has been reported in medical journals.[2]

Another family of toxins, called mutagens or carcinogens, can be produced from bacterial overgrowth in the intestines. Certain bac-

teria in the gut make dietary proteins and fats into unusual cancer-causing substances. If exposure to these types of toxins continues over time, cancer of the colon may develop. By restoring
the balance of bacteria in the gut and changing the diet, exposure
to this type of toxin can be reduced dramatically.

Sometimes we become so toxic from a combination of bacterial endotoxins, environmental chemicals and metabolic waste products that our systems of elimination become overloaded and cannot
keep up. In the process, our immune systems become sluggish.
When confronted with an infectious bacteria or virus, we simply
cannot muster adequate defenses to defeat it.

Parasites Lurking About

Another environmental cause of suppressed immunity is brought
about by intestinal parasites. Most of us probably view parasitic
infection as something only associated with Third World countries.
While it used to be true that parasite infections in the West were
uncommon, it is no longer the case. Names like *Giardia lamblia*
and *Entamoeba histolytica* are creeping into our everyday language
much like the names *Staphylococcus aureus* or *Streptococcus viridans*
(staph or strep). These organisms have made their way into our
water supply, food supply, day care centers and schools with growing frequency. Infection by these organisms is growing worldwide.

Chronic parasitic infection leads to poor digestion, development of allergies, nutrient malabsorption, fatigue and immune suppression. People with intestinal parasites often suffer from recurrent
bacterial and viral infections because of lowered immunity.

Timothy was a five-year-old boy who had experienced recurrent upper respiratory infections since birth. He had spent most
of his young life on antibiotics, with little improvement in health.
After further review of his history, it was discovered that Timothy's mother, an animal caretaker at a veterinarian's office, had
been infected with the parasite *Giardia lamblia* during her pregnancy. Yet, the pediatricians who cared for Timothy gave this no
consideration, convinced that antibiotics would resolve his recurrent
bronchial and ear infections. Timothy was finally tested and indeed
was infected with giardia. After treatment of the parasitic infec-

tion of the intestine and restoration of the normal ecology of the bowel, Timothy's recurrent upper respiratory infections were finally eliminated. Such intestinal infections commonly lead to suppressed immunity and generalized declines in health.

Heavy Metals and Immunity

Exposure to lead, mercury, cadmium, aluminum, nickel, arsenic and other metals can take a considerable toll on our immune systems. This can occur in infancy, childhood or adulthood. Metals can cause problems when present individually in high amounts. When more than one metal is present, which is often the case, even low levels can be damaging. This is because of a synergistic effect and the total toxic load. A recent study on prenatal exposure to heavy metals shows just how dramatic this effect can be.

Amniotic fluid was taken from 92 pregnant women and tested for the presence of seven heavy metals (cadmium, chromium, cobalt, lead, mercury, nickel and silver). A prenatal toxic risk score was assigned based on the presence and amount of the different heavy metals detected. This score was then correlated with the health of the children at age three. The researchers found that children with higher toxic risk scores *in utero* suffered from more infectious disease and allergies at age three than did children with low toxic risk scores. Listed in the category of infections were coughs, fever, sore throat, congestion, diarrhea, vomiting, ear infection and constipation. The authors of this paper wrote in *Pediatrics* in 1992, "The toxic risk score predicted the total number of illnesses and the number of infectious illnesses."*

The implications of this study are tremendous. If these children suffer from altered immunity as a result of toxic metal exposure, is it logical to treat their infectious episodes as mere bacterial invasion? Since we understand the importance of heavy metals in lowering immunity, should it not be routine practice to investigate the possibility of metal toxicity in all disorders involving immune function? Such questions should not be limited to childhood. As we

---

* Lewis, M., et al. Prenatal exposure to heavy metals. *Pediatrics* 1992; 89 (6): 1011–15

noted earlier, heavy metals affect immunity in people of all ages.

The presence of lead, mercury, cadmium, aluminum and other metals can take a considerable toll on our immune systems. When metals are identified and removed from the body, major improvements in well-being typically follow. Below is a discussion of the most important heavy metals, their sources and nutrients that are protective.

Mercury

Sources of mercury in the environment include dental amalgams (fillings that are mixtures of mercury, silver and other metals), some freshwater fish, shellfish, plastics, latex paint, DPT vaccine, organomercurial pesticides with fungicides, grains and seeds treated with methyl mercury or mercury chloride, and chlorine bleaches.

Nutrients that protect against mercury exposure include selenium, vitamin C, vitamin E, pectin, and the amino acids cysteine, cystine and methionine.

Lead

Common sources of lead include drinking water, lead dust from paint used in old homes, atmospheric pollution, leaded gasoline, lead-glazed pottery, wine and"tin cans" soldered with lead-containing solder. Canned tuna is a major source of lead in children.

The fall of the Roman empire (their water came from lead pipes and they drank from lead cups) and the demise of an entire race of Native Americans, the Omahas, are believed to be due to lead poisoning that slowly impaired the citizen's senses and destroyed their immune systems. Excavations of the skeletons of both nations showed high levels of lead in the bones, a common area of lead accumulation.

Nutrients that antagonize and protect against lead exposure include calcium, vitamin C, vitamin E, B-complex, pectin, and the amino acids cystine, cysteine and methionine.

Cadmium

Sources of cadmium include cigarette smoke, shellfish and other seafood, teas, paints, welding pigments, drinking water, galvanized pipes, batteries, auto exhaust, industrial smoke and waste. The processing of whole grains such as wheat into white flour strips off the zinc, a natural antagonist of cadmium, and leaves the cadmium to be sold to consumers.

Nutrients that protect against cadmium include zinc, vitamin C, selenium and to a limited extent, calcium.

Aluminum

Sources of aluminum include aluminum-containing antacids, aluminum-containing baking powder, aluminum antiperspirants, aluminum pots and pans, soft water, aluminum foil, DPT vaccine, and processed food containing aluminum.

Nutrients that protect against aluminum exposure include vitamin C, magnesium and calcium.

Arsenic

Sources of arsenic include tobacco smoke, smog, pesticides, caulks, glues and building materials that contain fungicides, beer, table salt, colored chalk and household laundry aids.

Nutrients that protect against arsenic include selenium and vitamin C.

No one can know for sure whether they have toxic metals in their system without testing. Hair analysis, despite the criticisms levied against it, is still considered one the most useful tests for screening for the presence of toxic metals in the body. Hair analysis is inexpensive and the sample easily taken. Tests of blood serum are only useful if the exposure has been recent. Tests of white blood cells and red blood cells are more useful than serum tests.

Urine tests are also very helpful in detecting the presence of toxic metals. First, a substance is given that chelates, or flushes, the metal from the system. The metal then shows up in the urine and can be measured. This test is usually done under a doctor's supervision. There are also new computer-based health questionnaires that indicate patterns of toxicity for the person taking the test.

Dental Amalgams: A Threat to Immunity?

There is growing concern among laypersons and health professionals about the potential hazards of mercury fillings. Mercury is undeniably a toxic metal that can have potentially devastating effects on immune function. Dental amalgams are a greater source of mercury exposure than any other non-occupational source.

Dr. Hal Huggins was one of the first to bring concern over the use of mercury in dental amalgams to public attention. Huggins has focused much of his work on the role of mercury leached from fillings in disrupting immune function. In 1985, he reported on the case of a man who had the mercury removed from his fillings. He writes, "We recently saw a patient with a white cell count of 235,000 (the medical normal is 5,000 to 10,000). After his amalgams had been out for only 40 hours there was a 60,000 count drop in total white cells. Other highly significant changes in the types of cells being produced to fight the infection in his body occurred during the same two-day period. He had arrived in our office on a Wednesday, certain that he would die of chronic myelogenous leukemia (CML) in three months. He returned to his home four days later, certain that he would live. Was he qualified to make this decision? Yes, he was a physician."[3]

Huggins and other dental colleagues have reported on a vast array of diseases and conditions, previously unresponsive to medical care, that improved following removal of mercury fillings. Patients suffering from multiple sclerosis, chronic fatigue syndrome, lupus, allergies, cardiovascular disease, kidney disease, depression, immunosuppressive disorders and other maladies have shown substantial improvement following removal of mercury from their teeth.

Recently, a new controversy has emerged surrounding the potential health hazards of mercury fillings. It appears that mercury from dental fillings can bring about changes in bacteria that cause them to be resistant to antibiotics. In a paper presented at the 1991 Annual Meeting of the American Society for Microbiology, Dr. A.O. Summers and colleagues reported on their study in which mercury fillings were placed in the mouths of monkeys. Various types of bacteria that live in the mouth and intestines were tested for resistance to antibiotics before and after placement of the fillings.

After installation of the fillings, investigators found a dramatic increase in bacterial resistance to multiple antibiotics including tetracycline, ampicillin, streptomycin, chloramphenicol and sulfadiazine. After five months, the mercury amalgam fillings were replaced by composite resin fillings that contained no mercury and the proportion of antibiotic-resistant bacteria declined. The researchers concluded that, "Constant exposure to Hg [mercury] arising from dental amalgams constitutes continuous selective pressure for the maintenance of multiply resistant bacteria in both oral and fecal flora of primates."[4] In other words, the fillings favored development of bacteria resistant to some of the most commonly used antibiotics in the medical arsenal.

The implications of this and other studies of mercury fillings and immune function are enormous. Is it possible that a vicious cycle is set in motion by the placement of amalgam fillings? Is it possible that the practice of using amalgams in dentistry seriously undermines the health of humans? Does this practice alter the fundamental nature of bacteria that live within our bodies? Presently there are a large number of studies that have begun to address such issues.

Even the attitude of dentists seem to be changing regarding amalgam safety. Years ago dentists concerned about the effects of amalgams on health were a distinct minority. In a 1990 survey, 6 percent of dentists did not use mercury amalgams and 39 percent were "concerned" or "highly concerned" about the safety of this filling material.[5]

If you suspect that mercury fillings might be contributing to poor health, you may wish to bring these concerns to the attention of a health professional who is knowledgeable in assessment and care of such problems. Another option is to contact the Environmental Dental Association (9974 Scripps Ranch Blvd., Suite 36, San Diego, CA 92131, 619-586-7626) or the Huggins Diagnostic Center (5080 List Drive, Colorado Springs, CO 80919, 800-331-2303) for more information.

The Electromagnetic Sea

As our society becomes more reliant upon electrical appliances and instruments, our exposure increases to what was once thought harmless forms of energy. Whenever an electrical motor is operated or electricity travels through a wire, an electromagnetic field is produced. Depending on certain factors such as amperage, wattage, frequency, wavelength and so on, the field can be projected great distances. For instance, the electromagnetic field produced by your television can project more than thirty feet and even travel through walls into the next room. The field from overhead power lines can project hundreds of feet into nearby homes. Radio waves and microwaves are projected nearly everywhere from towers high atop tall buildings. Exposure to both high-frequency and low-frequency electromagnetic waves is inescapable.

There is considerable debate over whether electromagnetic fields have an adverse effect on immune function. But a growing number of researchers are beginning to uncover a link that raises serious questions about how we will be able to manage immune system illness in the future. According to Robert O. Becker, M.D., leader in the study of the biological effects of electromagnetism, "Impaired immune response has been found at many frequencies. Several groups of Soviet researchers have found a decline in the efficiency of white blood cells in rats and guinea pigs after the animals had been exposed to radio waves and microwaves." Reporting on the work of one researcher, Becker writes ". . . the most dramatic effect on immune response has been produce by ELF [extremely low frequency] fields. Yuri N. Udintsev found that the concentration of bacteria needed to kill mice in such an environment was only one-fifth that needed without the field."[6]

Becker also reports in his book *The Body Electric* on the work of Yu N. Achkasova of the Crimean Medical Institute in Simferopol. Becker writes, "In 1978 they reported the results of exposing thirteen standard strains of bacteria—including anthrax, typhus, pneumonia, and staphylococcus—to electric and magnetic fields. After accounting for magnetic storms, ionospheric flux, passage of the interplanetary magnetic-field boundaries, and other variables, they found clear evidence that an electric field only slightly stronger than earth's background stimulated growth of all bacteria and increased their resistance to antibiotics. . . . Every field tested had an effect, even after one four-hour exposure. In many cases, longer exposure produced *permanent* changes in bacterial metabolism."[7]

It may be that with our technology we are altering the way in which our immune systems function *and* the virulence of organisms that live on this planet. If this work is verified by further research, it provides yet another strong argument for abandoning the "magic bullet" approach of allopathic medicine and concentrating our efforts on means of boosting immunity. It also suggests that we may need to look to our environment to answer some of our more puzzling medical questions.

Becker's recent book *Cross Currents: The Perils of Electropollution, The Promise of Electromedicine* (Jeremy P. Tarcher, 1990) looks at many aspects of electromagnetism—how it may cause disease and how, when used appropriately, it may cure disease.

Are You Exposed to Toxic Substances?

With regard to environmental toxins there is always a tendency to take an attitude of "it can't happen to me." But, the reality is that most of us are exposed on a daily basis, albeit to varying degrees. The National Academy of Sciences reports that an average American consumes roughly 40 milligrams of pesticides (DDT, DDE, DDD, etc.) each year in food alone and carries about 100 milligrams permanently in his or her body fat. Speaking on the subject of exposure to chemicals in our environment, Sherry Rogers, M.D., Fellow of the American Academy of Allergy and Immunology and a specialist in environmental medicine, sums it up quite succinctly. She states, "Even entering the world, most babies are already born with detectable levels of phthalates or plasticizers in their blood. It comes from the plastic in plastic bags and plastic I.V. tubing that was attached to the mothers before delivery. Studies have been done on people who just popped in the dry cleaner to pick up clothes. Four hours later they had measurable blood levels of perchloroethylene as opposed to negative levels in people who hadn't gone. Gassing up your car gives measurable benzene levels, drinking from a styrofoam cup gives measurable chemical levels."[8]

A simple example of how environmental chemicals flow through our body is found in cigarette smoke. Cotinine is a by-product of nicotine that is eliminated in the urine of smokers and people exposed to cigarette smoke. Only eight percent of infants in nonsmoking households show elevated levels of this chemical. In homes where one or both parents smoke, 96 percent of infants show elevated levels. Children of smoking parents suffer from more frequent respiratory infections, asthma and hospitalization than do other children. The chemicals found in cigarette smoke are known to contribute to this.[9]

One group of doctors analyzed the blood of 200 environmentally sensitive patients for 16 different synthetic compounds. An average of 3.4 chemical compounds was found per individual. The most common included hexachlorobenzene, heptachlorepoxide and members of the DDT family, dieldrin, beta-BHC and endosulfan 1. These are substances that didn't even exist 100 years ago, not to mention the fact that they are not a part of the body's normal metabolic machinery. That these compounds were found in the blood is surprising because the body usually tries to remove toxic substances from the blood and place them into other organs for storage. These findings suggest that even higher amounts were stored elsewhere in the body.[10]

So, are you exposed? Most of us are. How we respond depends upon our genetics, lifestyle, nutrition, exercise patterns, stress levels, attitudes and the level of substances to which we are exposed.

Is Your Building Making You Sick?

We noted earlier that the average person spends only one hour per day outdoors. This means roughly 23 hours a day are spent in the home, office or car. The stale air enclosed in these buildings is deficient in negative ions. It is also often filled with dust, mold, bacteria, particles and volatile substances that adversely influence our respiratory tract.

Three main factors have given rise to an increase in illness and complaints related to buildings. First, since the mid-1970s there has been a shift to more energy-efficient buildings. This has limited the amount of fresh air that circulates through homes, offices and schools. Second, there has been a dramatic increase in the use of synthetic building materials and furnishings. Most of these materials are made from petrochemicals that slowly release vapors over time (a process called outgassing). These vapors are known carcinogens and respiratory irritants. Finally, the proliferation of air-conditioned buildings has led to more bacterial and mold-related illness among people working in such places.

Offices with air conditioning typically produce the greatest number of complaints among office workers. According to an article in the *American Journal of Public Health,* air-conditioned buildings are "consistently associated with increased prevalence of work-related headache, lethargy, and upper respiratory/mucous membrane symptoms."[11]

Next on the list of symptom producers are *new* homes and offices. Jill was a healthy, 32-year-old real estate agent. She and her husband had planned many years and now eagerly awaited completion of their new "dream home." The move was uneventful. But after about two months, Jill began to complain of itchy eyes and nose, and a cough. After six months, she developed a severe cold that lasted about four months. Just over the cold, she developed tonsillitis. As time went on, she became more fatigued, weak, lethargic and seemed to come down with something every month or so. She received numerous different antibiotics in hopes that her recurrent illness might be cured, but the antibiotics further aggravated the situation. With more infections and antibiotics, she developed sensitivity to an ever-increasing number of foods. Jill was a victim of sick building syndrome—a reaction to the toxic vapors released by the glue, pressed wood, carpet, paint, varnish, furnishings and vinyl floor coverings used to build the home. This is an increasingly prevalent problem in modern times.

Use of chemicals within the home can also contribute to immune suppression. The case of Alex, aged two, is a classic example. Alex's parents were holistic physicians who took great pride in their own health practices. They transferred their diligence to their young son. Early in life Alex was quite healthy. Then, by some mystery, he began to develop chronic postnasal drip, stuffiness and middle ear fluid. None of these symptoms seemed to respond to any treatment. As they searched for answers, his parents realized that not long after they had sprayed their home for fleas—courtesy of the family pet—Alex's symptoms began. It was believed that the insecticides contained in the "flea bomb" suppressed Alex's immune system, which led to chronic problems. A similar situation occurred with Dr. Schmidt's mother, who developed chronic bronchitis and recurrent respiratory infections following treatment of her bedroom with "flea powder"—courtesy of the family dog!

Several years ago, and with great irony, workers at the office of the EPA (Environmental Protection Agency) were forced to move out of their new headquarters because of a flood of complaints of headache, nausea, burning eyes, fatigue and irritability. The culprits, formaldehyde and other volatile substances, were being released from building materials and paper supplies such as file folders. This certainly brought the issue of indoor air pollution to the fore.

Mold in the Home: Common Environmental Insult

Mold is something we usually associate with those dark spots lurking inside the shower curtain or perhaps that cheese that has spent too long in the refrigerator. Whatever the source, mold is an insidious culprit that can permeate the home and be a constant source of immune system stress. For some, the constant presence of mold in the home so heavily taxes the immune system on a daily basis that they easily succumb to opportunistic germs. Researchers in Canada recently reported that respiratory symptoms such as bronchitis and cough were much more common in homes where there was dampness or mold. Of the 15,000 homes studied, 32.4 percent reported mold, 21.4 percent reported flooding and 14.1 percent reported moisture from other causes.[12]

Air Pollution and Respiratory Infection

During the 1970s, we became acutely aware of the problems with air pollution and smog. Not much attention has been paid to these issues of late, which might lead us to believe the problem has improved. The unfortunate truth is that air quality in most major U.S. cities has gotten worse. Cases of asthma (and death from asthma) in children have been on the rise, as well as an increase in the rate of pneumonia among the elderly. Many doctors have attributed this in part to an increase in air pollutants.

According to a 1979 statement by the Surgeon General, "Increased air pollution has been associated with debilitating respiratory diseases such as acute and chronic bronchitis and pneumonia, and exacerbation [aggravation] of symptoms in people who already have pulmonary disease."

The most common air pollutants are sulfur dioxide, particulates, nitrogen oxide, hydrogen sulfide, and polycyclic aromatic hydrocarbons. These and other pollutants damage the lining of the respiratory tract and destroy the tiny hair-like cilia that are important for removal of bacteria, viruses, mold, pollen and particles. Once the respiratory tissues are damaged, we become susceptible to infection and allergy.

A classic example of the air pollution-infection link is illustrated by the outbreak of *Haemophilus influenzae* infections. This bacterium is known to contribute to many upper respiratory maladies, from ear infections to meningitis to bronchitis. Doctors write millions of antibiotic prescriptions each year in an effort to thwart this "virulent" organism. Yet, not everyone exposed to the germ becomes sick. Indeed, deaths from chronic bronchitis are 30 times more frequent in the United Kingdom than in the United States. What are the factors that influence susceptibility to this bug?

Bernard Dixon, Ph.D., sheds light on the matter of *Haemophilus influenzae* bronchitis when he states, "This has been termed the English disease, and the blame has been attached to the country's damp, inhospitable climate. Even that is not the full story. Within Britain, bronchitis is largely a town disease, being rare in rural areas but widespread in industrial centres. It is also an affliction of the poor; mortality is highest among unskilled men and women and falls progressively to reach its lowest level among professional people." He continues, "Thus the memorable events in the story of bronchitis are not major epidemics triggered by the emergence of especially virulent strains of bacteria. They are episodes of horrendous air pollution, caused by the engines of industry, which kill people already suffering from the disease. One such episode occurred at Donora, south of Pittsburgh, in 1948, when there was a major fog and weather inversion. By the third day of the four-day incident, over 40 percent of the people in Donora, a town in a river valley surrounded by hills, were affected by respiratory illness, with cough, sore throat, nasal discharge, smarting of the eyes, tears, nausea, headache, weakness and occasional muscle aches and pains."[13]

If you live in an area with poor air quality (Los Angeles, San Francisco, New York City, Detroit and many others), you probably need to increase your intake of vitamins C and E, beta-carotene and selenium. Each of these play an essential role in protecting our cell linings from airborne pollutants. You also may consider moving, or using an air filter in the home (although this will only make a small impact).

Exposure on the Job

Some occupations are at particular risk for exposure to toxic chemicals. Examples include farmers, hair stylists, professional painters, chemists, miners, floor installers, manufacturing technicians, auto mechanics, dry cleaning workers, custodians, contractors, print shop operators and so on. If you work in one of these occupations (or any occupation that uses synthetic chemicals) and suffer from chronic or recurrent health problems (or infections), chances are that your body is toxic. This may be having an adverse effect on your immune system, making you susceptible to a variety of germs. You should be especially suspicious if you suffer from vague complaints that your doctors can't seem to understand or treat.

Ken was a farmer from southern Minnesota. One day he was loading seed corn into the corn planter in preparation for spring planting, a ritual he had performed for years. On this fateful day he squatted down to pick up the open bag of seed corn. As he wrapped his arms around the bag, a huge "puff" of red powder was forced from the bag, just as Ken was inhaling deeply. He coughed and began to feel dizzy. Shortly thereafter he noticed blood in his urine. After several hours his urine had become pure crimson due to the high number of red blood cells being spilled into his urine. He was taken to Mayo Clinic. The red powder to which Ken was exposed was mercury chloride, a commonly used fungicide. Ken had elevated levels of mercury in his tissues and began to experience kidney, neurologic and immune problems. His doctors at Mayo Clinic were unable to offer any assistance. Ken's problems improved only after going through a detoxification program provided by his chiropractic physician.

If you work in an occupation that uses any solvents, cleaning compounds, paints, pesticides, herbicides, lawn care chemicals, varnishes, printer's ink, dry cleaning supplies, hair care products, plastics or textiles, you may have exposure to low levels of toxics. If there are any unusual smells in your workplace or home, they usually represent some sort of toxic substance in the air. In either case, you should consider being evaluated for toxic chemical exposure and/or going through detoxification or metabolic clearing therapy.

Pollutants Cause Malnourishment

One insidious effect of exposure to chemicals in our environment is the loss or destruction of nutrients in our bodies. Loss of nutrients renders us more susceptible to harm by subsequent exposure to these and other chemicals in the future. For example, vitamin B_6 is essential for the enzymes that detoxify the toxic substance toluene. Yet, B_6 can be antagonized by exposure to this and other toxic substances, making the job of detoxication* much more difficult. Moreover, nutrients antagonized by toxic exposure, such as vitamins A and C and the mineral zinc, are critical to optimum function of the immune system. Consider only a few examples cited in a chapter entitled "Environmental Medicine" published in *The Kellogg Report,* by Joseph Beasley, M.D.:[14]

- Workers handling pesticides suffer from severe disruption of vitamin A.

- Exposure to even low levels of PCBs cuts the vitamin A stored in the liver of animals by 50 percent.

- Deficiency of vitamin E worsens the ill effects of nitrogen dioxide from smog.

- More than 20 cigarettes per day lowers blood levels of vitamin C by 40 percent.

Nutrients have also been used to protect against pollutants and to treat exposure. For example:

---

*The term *detoxication* is usually used to describe the body's own mechanism for handling toxic substances. *Detoxification* refers to a therapeutic process used to rid the body of toxins.

- Zinc reduces liver damage by the chemical solvent carbon tetrachloride.

- Selenium and vitamin E protect against lung damage by ozone.

- In workers exposed to toxic fluorine, vitamin C enabled the body to excrete the toxin more rapidly.

In Chapter 4, we discussed the adverse effects prescription drugs can have on nutritional status. It appears that prescription drugs also influence our bodily response to pollutants. Tagamet® is one of the most widely prescribed prescription drugs in the United States. There is evidence that this and other drugs can serve to intensify the toxicity of pesticides to which one might be exposed. This evidently happens because the drugs disrupt liver function. Efficient liver function is crucial to the rapid elimination of toxins.[15,16]

A "Good Diet" Is Not Enough

Most patients who have asked their doctor to recommend a vitamin or mineral supplement are rebuffed with, "Vitamin and mineral supplements aren't necessary. Just eat a good diet and you'll get all the nutrients you need." This thinking defies logic. First, no one is sure of what a "good diet" really is. Even when we eat whole grains, fruits, vegetables, lean meat or fish, etc., can we really be sure we are getting all the nutrients we need? An orange loses 50 percent of its vitamin C 24 hours after harvest. Yet, by the time you eat it, it may have spent weeks or months in a warehouse. Food transport and storage have made our lives more convenient, but we may be paying a price in nutrient content.

Exposure to so many substances in our environment has changed the ground rules for living in the twenty-first century. As evidence mounts, it is becoming clear that nutrient amounts beyond what we get in our daily food may be necessary to merely cope with the daily exposure to foreign chemicals. Optimum health may require even greater nutrient amounts depending on our diet, lifestyle and degree of exposure. This is especially true for the antioxidant nutrients A, E, C, beta-carotene and selenium.

Signs of a Toxic Body

The signs of a toxic body do not fit neatly into any diagnostic category. This is often why allopathic doctors fail to recognize or consider such symptoms. In general, symptoms of toxicity are very vague and broad. Fatigue, sluggishness and just a low level of wellness are hallmarks. Common symptoms of toxicity include:

- Fatigue
- Lethargy
- Depression
- Headaches
- Allergies
- Muscle aches
- Chronic infections
- Frequent colds
- Sluggishness
- Nervousness, irritability
- Sensitivity to perfume, odors
- Joint pains

Reducing Toxins in Your Body

For many years it was thought that once chemicals such as toluene, PCBs or DDT were lodged in our bodies, it was impossible to remove them. Fortunately, new approaches have been developed that help us to reduce the toxic load in our tissues. In *Human & Experimental Toxicology* it was shown that detoxification techniques reduced the amount of toxins by 63 percent in the body of a woman poisoned with PCBs.[17]

Jeffrey S. Bland, Ph.D., one of the leading researchers and educators in the field of nutritional biochemistry, has recently pioneered a detoxification program that significantly improves the elimination of toxins. He reports that certain individuals who suffer from chronic or recurrent infections (and other problems) have an elevated toxic load that adversely affects function of the immune system. In order for the immune system to function normally in these people, the toxic load must be reduced or eliminated.[18] The following case illustrates this point.

Ellen was a 40-year-old executive vice president of a growing Minneapolis company. She suffered from repeated bladder and upper respiratory infections that were treated with antibiotics.

Vaginal infections often followed. She suffered from extreme fatigue that caused her to leave work early several days a week. Some days she was unable to go to work. She experienced frequent headaches, muscle aches, intestinal bloating and insomnia. Ellen commonly felt depressed and unhappy about life.

Ellen was placed on a detoxification program using UltraClear® developed by Dr. Bland and used in many clinics nationwide. The plan consisted of consuming foods unlikely to provoke allergic reactions (rice, squash, pears, organic chicken, broccoli, etc.) while drinking a mixture of UltraClear® and juice or water three times daily. The total duration of the cleanse was 14 days. During the first few days of the cleanse, Ellen felt somewhat "foggy" and tired. Gradually, her energy returned. Most of the symptoms she reported had resolved. She continued to take UltraClear® twice weekly for three months and continued to improve. Ellen was able to return to her normal work schedule with little difficulty.

This case is only one of many accounts of people with lowered immunity who have benefited from detoxification or cleansing programs. If you suspect environmental factors may have diminished your level of health and well-being, it may be necessary to consult a doctor who is knowledgeable in environmental medicine, nutrition and detoxification.

Testing for Toxic Exposure

Numerous tests are now being developed that will help determine whether we've been exposed to toxic substances and how significant that exposure is to our health. Two such tests in use today can be part of an important first step in assessing whether toxic exposure has impaired your health. The first test is known as D-glucaric acid. This is a test that measures whether you've been exposed to toxic chemicals. It does not specify which chemical, however. D-glucaric acid is performed on a urine specimen that is collected over a 24-hour period. Your doctor can order this for you.

Another useful test is urinary mercapturic acid. This substance is an actual by-product of the normal detoxication process of the body. If mercapturic acid levels in the urine are high, you have been exposed to foreign chemicals. This test also is performed on a 24-hour urine specimen. (MetaMetrix Medical Research Laboratory, Norcross, Georgia 30071)

Your doctor can perform both the mercapturic acid and D-glucaric acid tests to determine your level of toxic exposure. Using these tests, researchers have been able to differentiate between office and industrial plant workers by the level of mercapturic acid and D-glucaric acid in their urine. Those working in offices have lower levels of these compounds in their urine compared with co-workers in the manufacturing section of the same plant.

Another useful test is the caffeine clearance test (MetaMetrix). A small amount of caffeine is ingested. Saliva samples are then measured to determine how efficiently the liver eliminates the substance. If high levels of caffeine remain in the saliva it means the liver is functioning poorly and suggests the need for some kind of detoxification therapy. Remember, the liver is the primary organ responsible for eliminating toxic substances from the body. If it is not functioning properly, even small amounts of a substance can be detrimental.

A useful blood test is called the ELISA/ACT test (Serammune Physicians Lab, 1890 Preston White Drive, Suite 200, Reston VA 22091, 800-553-5472). This test is helpful in identifying immune reactivity to environmental chemicals such as pesticides, herbicides, food additives and other products.

The Low-Temperature Sauna: Powerful Detoxifier

Saunas are being used by some doctors to stimulate the release of toxins from the bodies of their patients. They have found that a lower-temperature (105°–110° F) sauna taken for a longer duration (45–90 minutes a day for several weeks) is most beneficial. These low temperatures stimulate a fat sweat, which eliminates toxins stored in fat, as opposed to the high-temperature sauna, which encourages a water sweat.

The principle is summed up as follows: "The body's fat must be warmed to increase its solubility; the warmed fat must be transportable to the sweat glands which excrete fat; the process must continue long enough for appreciable 'fat sweat' to occur; the temperature must be low enough that the person does not lose significant amounts of water or electrolytes; the sweat oils must be vigorously washed off. We find glycerine soaps (such as Neutrogena, Black Soap, and similar 'super-fatted' soaps) the most effective here. Use of a loofah as a gentle scrub brush is also helpful."[19]

The low-temperature sauna is usually carried out 5 to 7 days a week for three months and then 3 days a week for three months. (This should be done under a doctor's supervision. Our discussion of it here is meant only to show the value of the procedure.) In addition, nutrients are given that help to bind the toxins or minimize their effect on the body. Included are B-vitamins, vitamins C, E and beta-carotene and trace minerals such as zinc, magnesium, calcium and selenium. Using this method, doctors have been able to measure toxic compounds released in the sweat of their patients. These chemicals are often toxic to the immune system, nervous system, endocrine system and liver. "Sweating them out" reduces chemical stress on the body and generally leads to improved health.

Physician and researcher, Zane R. Gard, M.D. (P.O. Box 1791, Beaverton, Oregon 97075), has developed a detoxification regimen known as the BioToxic Reduction™ Program (BTR). This program has been used with great success in managing toxicity due to drugs and environmental poisons. His approach incorporates the use of a carefully regulated sauna along with massage, exercise, nutritional supplements, psychological counseling, and daily doses of oils that help draw toxins out of the intestinal tract. This program was initiated in 1983 and has many case histories, statistics and laboratory data affirming its effectiveness.

A Strategy for Living in Modern Times

We've shown that virtually everyone comes in contact with toxic substances on a daily basis. It is unavoidable. Since we cannot eliminate these substances from our world we must do the next best things:

1. Try to reduce our exposure.
2. Periodically eliminate toxins from our bodies.
3. Ensure that we take extra nutrients that are helpful in combating exposure to these chemicals and minimizing their impact.

We can reduce our exposure by limiting the amount of synthetic substances we use directly, such as cleaning compounds, nail polish, paints and varnishes, lawn care chemicals, and so on. The books *Non-Toxic and Natural* and *The Non-Toxic Home* by Deborah Lynn Dadd contain a detailed description of alternatives that are also more compatible with the environment.

Above, we described a detoxification program to eliminate toxins from our bodies. Such programs are usually used with people who have chronic illness, recurrent infections, known exposure to toxic substances, or non-specific complaints that befuddle their doctors. However, because of the constant exposure to low levels of thousands of man-made chemicals on a daily basis, many doctors now recommend that people go through a periodic cleanse, perhaps every six months. This helps reduce the total toxic load on our bodies and the untoward effects that might follow.

This recommendation has numerous historical precedents. Ancient traditions have for centuries recommended periods of fasting to cleanse the body and the soul. We now have definitive scientific proof that such cleansings are vital to our health. Most recently, however, we have learned that a true fast, in which nothing is eaten, wastes muscle. A cleanse in which a supply of calories and nutrients is provided is more sound.

A final solution to living in a toxic world is to take antioxidant nutrients on a daily basis. The importance of taking adequate vitamin C is described in Chapter 8. Other nutrients vital to our detoxication processes are magnesium, zinc, selenium, vitamin E and beta-carotene. Extracts of milk thistle *(Silybum marianum)* seed are being used extensively to protect the body from toxic exposure and to repair damaged liver tissue when toxic exposure has occurred. More than 200 clinical and laboratory studies have shown that the active constituent in milk thistle, silymarin, is one of the most potent liver-protecting substances known. We have used this to treat patients who have environmental illness, who have been exposed to toxic substances or who must be on drugs that are toxic to the liver. It has even been helpful in reversing cases of alcohol-induced cirrhosis of the liver. Silymarin is also a potent antioxidant.

Note: Pregnant women should not undergo detoxification because toxins released from fat stores can expose the fetus.

A Summary of Things to Do

1. Limit your use of synthetic materials.

2. Sauna regularly to help purge toxic compounds from your body.

3. Do a periodic cleansing of your internal body using the Metabolic Clearing Therapy or some variation. Many with sluggish immune systems experience dramatic improvement following such programs. Even those who are not ill experience a heightened sense of well-being.

4. If you suffer from chronic or recurrent infections, you may be toxic. Have an evaluation done by a doctor familiar with environmental medicine. Certain blood and urine tests can detect exposure to toxins you may not be aware of.

5. If you work in an occupation in which chemicals are used, have regular check-ups and consider having blood and urine analysis to detect toxic exposure. It may be especially important that you do a cleanse.

6. Avoid synthetic personal hygiene products.

7. Take extra antioxidant nutrients including vitamins C and E, beta-carotene and selenium. Also use zinc and magnesium.

8. Use liver-protecting herbs such as milk thistle seed extract.

9. Drink water purified by carbon filtration and reverse osmosis, especially if you live in an area with landfills or known chemical contaminants.

10. Wear protective gloves and clothing whenever working with toxic chemicals at home or at work. This includes common lawn and garden products.

6

Heredity and Lifestyle

"Like the food we eat and the environment that pervades us, our personal behavior—or lifestyle—plays a fundamental role in shaping our health."

Joseph D. Beasley, M.D.
The Institute of Health Policy and Practice[1]

Most medical experts now agree that the major causes of death today—cancer, heart disease, stroke, etc.—are related to lifestyle and habits. There is strong evidence that modification of these habits results in substantial improvements in health and a decline in the number of deaths due to these illnesses. Though the "experts" recognize this, they have not extended their thinking to include common infectious conditions for which antibiotics are routinely given. Immunity and resistance to infections are clearly responsive to changes in lifestyle and habits. By making practical use of knowledge currently available, we can help reduce the incidence of infectious diseases and further reduce our reliance on antibiotic drugs.

Is it in Your Genes?

Genes play a crucial role in determining our individual make-up. From hair color to eye and skin color, the genes determine our basic appearance. Genes also influence specific metabolic needs at the cellular level. The fundamental machinery that drives every biochemical process in the body is similar in everyone, but there are vast differences in efficiency and needs among individuals.

In a massive undertaking to map the human genome, scientists have learned that even though a gene for a specific tendency, disease or condition may exist, its expression is subject to environmental factors. The environment referred to here is both the external and the nutritional environment. For instance, carriers of a particular gene are predisposed to the development of rectal polyps that develop into benign tumors and eventually colon cancer. These people have 14 times the risk of developing colorectal cancer than the average person. When such patients were given vitamin C (4 g/day), vitamin E (400 IU/day), and a grain fiber supplement (22.5 g/day), the development of these polyps was stopped. Presumably their risk of developing colon cancer was reduced as well.[2] This study suggests that such patients have metabolic needs very different from those we consider to be "average." Likewise, carriers of a gene that predisposes to lung cancer might be able to prevent the expression of that gene, i.e., lung cancer, by not smoking and by consuming more vitamin A, beta-carotene and vitamin C. It was unheard of decades ago to think that a genetic condition could be modified by nutritional means.

Another example of the genetic link is children with Down syndrome, who suffer from more frequent infections (usually treated with antibiotics) than do other children. While no one is likely to suggest that Down syndrome can be reversed, there are certain "expressions" associated with Down syndrome that can be modified with nutrition. Recently it was found that children with Down syndrome have a defect in an enzyme that makes them more susceptible to the ravages of free-radicals. This makes their need greater for antioxidant nutrients such as vitamins C and E. Some immune deficiency problems experienced by Down syndrome children can be reversed by zinc supplementation.

Children with Down syndrome are especially prone to respiratory bacterial infection, evidently because they do not make enough antibodies to fight the bacteria most commonly found in upper respiratory infections—*Haemophilus influenzae* and *Streptococcus pneumoniae*. When these children are given the trace element selenium, antibodies against these bacteria increase and the frequency of respiratory infections goes down.[3]

People with a genetic condition called Chediak-Higashi disease suffer from severe infections that occur because their white blood cells do not respond normally. It was shown over 15 years ago that increasing the intake of vitamin C protects these people against infection. It does not correct the underlying genetic fault, but some effects of the disease are rectified.[4]

These genetic conditions do not affect the majority of individuals. However, intolerance to the milk sugar lactose and the cow's milk protein casein are common and familiar to many of us. These genetically determined conditions can result in trouble ranging from chronic digestive difficulty to recurrent tonsillitis. Those who are affected by these problems improve their health by avoiding the offending agents.

Allergy can also be inherited. The term "atopy" is used to describe a common inherited predisposition to develop allergy. If both parents are atopic, there is a 75 percent chance that a child will have allergic symptoms. If one parent has atopy, the child has a 50 percent chance. Atopy can set the stage for recurrent infections of the ear, nose and bronchial tract by creating a mucus-rich environment for the invasion and multiplication of bacteria, viruses or yeast. Atopy itself is not treated with antibiotics, but some of the complications, such as ear infections, are treated with antibiotics. Atopic individuals have been shown to have a defect in an enzyme system that influences inflammation and immunity. By altering the diet and supplementing with specific vitamins, minerals and essential fatty acids, the problems associated with this condition can be reduced for many sufferers.

One way to understand the importance of genetics in our susceptibility to disease is to look at twins. Identical twins—derived from the same egg who share the same genes—have uniquely similar resistance to infection. If one identical twin has the clinical disease tuberculosis, the other twin has roughly a 75 percent chance of developing it as well. In contrast, a non-identical twin has only a 33 percent chance of developing the disease.[5] Racial differences are revealing as well. Pneumonia, rheumatic fever and tuberculosis are much more prevalent and severe in African-Americans than in those of European heritage.

Even hair color may have an indirect association with infection susceptibility. It is a well-known but poorly understood phenomenon that red-haired people have a tendency toward hypothyroidism. Those with low thyroid function are unusually susceptible to infection by bacteria and viruses. According to Stephen E. Langer, M.D., "I had never seen a naturally red-haired person who was not at least slightly hypothyroid. . . . An auburn-haired person who is not hypothyroid is a rare bird."*

Such examples underscore the fact that each of us is individually unique. While our genetic makeup may not render us seriously impaired, there are differences in each of us. Your need for a certain vitamin or mineral may be greater than that of your neighbor. Your immune system may require greater amounts of a substance in order to function optimally. This concept of biochemical individuality was advanced in great depth by pioneering researcher Roger Williams, formerly at the University of Texas.

Dr. Williams spent many years studying animals thought to be genetically uniform. To his surprise (and that of the scientific community), the body chemistry of these animals varied widely. According to Dr. Williams, "Early in our experience, especially after we became interested in biochemical individuality, my coworkers and I observed many disparities among those supposedly uniform animals. Some inbred rats on identical diets excreted eleven times as much urinary phosphate as others; some when given a chance to exercise at will, ran consistently twenty times as far as others; some voluntarily consumed consistently sixteen times as much sugar as others; some drank twenty times as much alcohol; some appeared to need about forty times as much vitamin A as others; some young guinea pigs required for good growth at least twenty times as much vitamin C as others."[6,7,8] Dr. Williams' work has been confirmed in humans.

Whether one is right—or left-handed also appears to have influence on immunity. While handedness is not necessarily a genetic trait, there is evidence that it has familial origins. Studies have now shown that individuals who are left-handed suffer from immune disorders at nearly three times the rate of their right-handed counterparts.[9]

---

*Langer, SE, Scheer, JF. *Solved: the riddles of illness,* New Canaan, Connecticut: Keats Publishing, 1984;39.

So what is our point in discussing these issues? Medicine has spent much of its time studying what some refer to as "statistical humans." Statistics tries to find averages and norms and tries to fit everybody into some sort of category. It does not take into account the differences in each of us. Doctors often admonish us to "eat a normal diet." But how do they know if that diet is best for you—supposing there is such a thing as a normal diet. If your need for vitamin C is 10 times the average, you will only experience good health if your need is met. If your need for zinc is twice the average, you will eventually become ill if you receive less. If you are genetically inclined to deficiencies in immune function, you might suffer from infections until your nutritional optimum is found. It is really quite exciting, for we will increasingly have the means to improve health by specifically providing what each individual needs. So remember, although genes are important, we are not hostages to our genes. They make us who we are. But recognize that you are unique, and strive to find a diet and lifestyle that optimize your ability to be well!

A Legacy for Our Children

Doctors have known for some time that the dietary habits and nutritional status of a pregnant mother affect her unborn offspring. Poor nutrition can lead to prematurity, developmental delays, learning difficulties and immune deficiency. Dr. Lucille Hurley and her co-workers at the University of California at Davis looked at the impact of parental nutritional status on offspring. To do this, they placed pregnant mice on a moderately zinc-deficient diet and observed for changes in immune function. The first-generation offspring (F1) showed depressed immune function as a result of the parents' low-zinc diet. Remarkably, the next two generations of mice (F2 and F3) also experienced lowered immune function *despite the* fact that they and the parents were fed a diet containing normal levels of zinc.[10]

There also seem to be genetic implications if the parents do not consume adequate amounts of vitamin C. It seems that low levels of vitamin C can lead to genetic damage in sperm. Dr. Bruce Ames at the University of California at Berkeley found that men who were fed diets low in vitamin C (10 or 20 mg per day) experienced more damage to the DNA in their sperm than those who consumed higher amounts of vitamin C. Such damage to DNA could potentially lead to genetic disorders, birth defects, immune deficiency or cancer in children.[11]

If the work of Drs. Hurley and Ames is true, it would suggest that the dietary choices of your parents have the potential to affect both you and your children. Your children's immune competence may in turn be affected by your dietary choices. This is of great concern given the poor dietary habits of many people in the United States. For instance, the levels of zinc and essential fatty acids, both necessary for proper immune function, do not even meet the very conservative RDA in almost half of all nursing mothers. Most infant formulas contain little or none of the important fatty acids needed for development of the brain and immune system. Many people consume less than optimum amounts of vitamin C. This is especially true of those who smoke. It is also true of all who must live in an increasingly polluted world. A 1982 report showed that 78 percent of (76) healthy pregnant American women had one or more *glaring* vitamin deficiencies.[12]

What impact does this have on the immune competence of our children? Is it a coincidence that the occurrence of ear infections, bronchial infections, meningitis, allergies, parasitic infection, asthma and other childhood disorders is on the rise? Couple poor parental nutrition with poor infant and childhood nutrition and one can imagine why these problems have emerged. Add to this the overuse of antibiotics, which further disrupts intestinal ecology and nutrient assimilation, and one is led to believe that the riddle of the increase in such illness will not be solved until doctors adopt a more holistic view of health.

Hygiene, Lifestyle and Personal Habits

According to physician and epidemiologist Thomas McKeown, the factor perhaps most responsible for the dramatic decline in infectious disease was improvement in hygiene—both personal and public. In his book *The Role of Medicine* he points out that "The largest contribution of biomedical science was the extension of hygiene measures" and that "control of infections resulted mainly from modification of the conditions under which they occurred."[13] Tremendous improvements in our resistance to disease can be made by modifying our lifestyle, habits and hygiene. Below are numerous factors important to boosting immunity and preventing infection.

Turn Up the Heat

Perhaps one of today's most overlooked hygienic practices for improving health is the use of saunas and steambaths. These have been used by people from many cultures for centuries. Virtually all of the Indians of North America used steambaths. According to anthropologist Jack Weatherford, "The widespread and persistent use of the steambaths and of the water baths by the Indians paralleled the practices of ancient Mediterranean cultures, but stood in sharp contrast to the practice of the Europeans who arrived in the New World. *The bathing probably served to reduce disease among the Indians prior to the European arrival and thereby partly accounted for the general freedom from epidemic diseases. The destruction of the lodges by the Europeans and their denunciation of frequent bathing quite probably contributed to the rapid spread of Old World epidemics among the natives of North America.*" [emphasis added][14]

Steambaths and saunas are also a well-known component of the Finnish repertoire of healthy living. The Finnish people have long contended that weekly saunas are an essential part of preventing disease and living a long life. They also serve as a kind of social encounter in which families and friends gather to share stories, laugh and play.

But is there a scientific basis to these beliefs about the benefits of saunas and steambaths? The answer appears to be "yes." German researchers recently studied 22 kindergarten children who partook of a weekly sauna and compared them with a control group who took no saunas. The children were followed for 18 months and a careful record was made of their incidence of ear infections, colds and other upper respiratory problems. Children who took no saunas suffered from *twice* the number of sick days as their steamier counterparts. The conclusion: children who sauna regularly have an improved resistance to infections.[15] The same probably holds true for adults.

In 1992, Dr. Schmidt interviewed members of a Minnesota health club as they exited the sauna. Many reported that the number of colds, sinus infections, bouts with the flu and bronchial infections went down or became non-existent after they began to sauna regularly. One man remarked, "I used to get sinus infections that typically lasted the entire winter. Since I take a sauna every week or so, I rarely ever get an infection." In the midst of one of the nastiest epidemics of influenza in recent memory, another man stated, "My wife was sick for nine days and I thought I was next. I felt the same symptoms coming on and took a 20-minute sauna for each of the next four days. That did it. I never got sick!"

Frequent use of steambaths or saunas probably helps reduce infections by stimulating profuse perspiration that enhances elimination of metabolic toxins from the body while also raising body temperature. Elevated body temperature (fever) is a common means used by the body to wage war with microbes of all types. In fact, one expert has called fever "Mother Nature's best antibiotic!"

Another practice that has survived the ages is vigorous rubbing of the skin in the bath, shower or sauna. This helps remove old dead skin, stimulates circulation and aids in the elimination of toxins. The skin is the largest organ of elimination in the entire body. Dr. Sehnert tells his patients, "Your skin is like a *third kidney*—it constantly gets rid of toxins of all kinds." When we treat the skin well and make use of its inherent cleansing abilities, we put the odds for good health on our side!

Light and the Immune Response

The average person in our Western world spends less than one hour daily outdoors. We sleep in darkness, awaken indoors to artificial light, drive to work in a car, toil for eight hours under artificial fluorescent light, complete our work, drive home, eat dinner indoors and go to bed. Depending on the day of the week or the season, we may get a few hours outdoors. But generally, we're short on natural light.

In contrast, our predecessors of 100 years ago spent the bulk of their day outdoors. Artificial light had nowhere near the impact it does today. There is now evidence that the absence of light experienced by most of us exacts a measurable toll on our mood, behavior, productivity and general level of health.

In some people, absence of adequate sunlight leads to development of a condition called seasonal affective disorder, or SAD. This condition is characterized by lethargy, fatigue, depression, insomnia and irritability. It is most pronounced during the winter months—especially in northern climates where it has been called "cabin fever." Sufferers respond dramatically to daily exposure to full-spectrum light. These people have found by trial and error that a winter week in Florida, Arizona or the Caribbean dramatically improves their outlook on life.

SAD is not the only condition that responds to sunlight. We've known for decades that treatment of jaundiced babies with blue light results in a rapid elimination of excess bilirubin from the body (full-spectrum lights work even better).

Light is as vital to our health as vitamins and minerals. In fact, the manufacture of vitamin D is actually dependent upon adequate exposure to ultraviolet light from the sun. We are only beginning to discover the many bodily processes that are dependent upon daily exposure to natural light. Whether light actually enhances immune function or increases resistance to disease is another question. However, recent reports suggest that light plays a role in these vital functions as well.

German researcher Dr. Fritz Hollwich discovered that when subjects sat under standard cool-white fluorescent lights, the levels of ACTH and cortisol (stress hormones) rose to levels comparable to those found in people under stress. In contrast, those sitting under full-spectrum light experienced no such rise in stress hormones. High levels of these hormones are known to have an adverse effect upon immune function. In view of this research, German hospitals are no longer allowed to use cool-white fluorescent bulbs.[16]

It was recently found that switching from cool-white fluorescent lights to full-spectrum lights reduced the number of workplace absences due to illness. Based on this and other evidence, some doctors suggest that full-spectrum light boosts immune function much like natural sunlight.

Studies in Germany and Russia suggest that providing adequate ultraviolet light can be useful in managing infectious diseases in schools and in the workplace.[17,18,19] In one study conducted in the 1940s, modifying environmental factors such as lighting in the classroom of school children resulted in a 43.3 percent reduction in the incidence of chronic infections.[20]

A Sneeze and a Handshake

How does illness spread from one person to another? The answer depends upon which illness and which microorganism you look at. In his book *Cold Cures,* author Michael Castleman reviews the debate that has waged over how common cold viruses are transmitted. Citing numerous research studies that have sought to answer the question, Castleman concludes that airborne droplets serve as the route of transmission for a percentage of viruses while hand-to-hand contact is the vehicle for others. Viruses are deposited on the hands while blowing or picking one's nose or by sneezing. The viruses are then passed to others via handshakes or contact with inanimate objects that are later touched by unsuspecting victims.

Likewise, bacteria can be spread by either airborne routes or by contact. In addition, some are spread via the fecal-oral route, contaminated food or contaminated water.

Castleman recommends the following to prevent the transmission of colds:[21]

1. Wash your hands frequently with soap and water, especially if you or a housemate or workmate suffer from a cold.
2. Keep your hands away from your nose and eyes. Nose pickers are more prone to upper respiratory infections.
3. Use disposable facial tissue, not cloth handkerchiefs.
4. Disinfect children's toys and household and workplace objects and surfaces with Lysol.
5. Try to stay home for the first day or two of cold symptoms—when virus shedding peaks.

Researchers in Japan have recently discovered that toothbrushes act as a breeding ground for some very pesky germs. When they examined the toothbrushes of 150 children they observed that most contained over one million bacteria! A thorough rinsing of the toothbrush only cut the number of bacteria in half.[22] Thus, the toothbrush may be a source of transmission of germs among families. A solution is to thoroughly clean the toothbrush with soap and water followed by hydrogen peroxide after someone has been ill. Replace toothbrushes every two to three months.

These recommendations can be helpful in preventing the spread of other contagious illnesses as well. Remember, while colds are not due to bacterial infections, they commonly lead to conditions such as earaches and bronchitis, which are often treated with antibiotics.

Where There's Smoke There's . . . Illness

Information about the adverse health effects of cigarette smoke is nothing new. We know those who smoke are more likely to develop heart disease, lung cancer and a variety of other ills. The negative effects of second-hand smoke are receiving more attention lately. In fact, the EPA has recently listed second-hand cigarette smoke as a carcinogen (cancer-causing agent).

Beyond its ability to cause cancer, second-hand smoke serves as a respiratory irritant that can contribute to recurrent ear, bronchial and sinus infections. Kids who live in homes with smokers have up to a four-fold greater risk of developing middle ear infections than kids who live in homes without smokers. Hospitalization for respiratory illness is also higher among those who live in homes with smokers.

Cigarette smoke causes excessive amounts of vitamin C to be eliminated from the body and increases the need for other nutrients such as vitamin E and beta-carotene. In a recent study, only one-third of smokers consumed enough vitamin C to meet the very conservative RDA. Moreover, the smokers required over twice as much vitamin C daily to achieve the same amount of vitamin C in the blood as nonsmokers.[23]

If there's a smoker in the house, do one of two things: get them to quit or have them smoke outside the home. Also, for second-hand smoke take at least 250 to 1,000 mg of vitamin C, 200 IU of vitamin E and 25,000 IU of beta-carotene daily. If you smoke and choose not to quit, take at least 1,000 to 2,000 mg of vitamin C,

400 IU of vitamin E and 50,000 IU of beta-carotene daily. *Your* health may depend upon it!

Do Couch Potatoes Suffer More Illness?

This is a difficult question to answer. People who watch hours of TV tend to snack more, eat more junk food, exercise less, and to be more sedentary and overweight. These factors may influence nutritional status to the extent that immunity is impaired—but no one is certain. Another problem is that constant TV viewing causes fatigue, emotional exhaustion and irritability. Viewers generally feel more anxiety after watching TV than before. In addition, both children and adults who watch a lot of TV tend to view the world as a more hostile and violent place than those who watch little or no TV.

TV-viewing couch potatoes pay another price—obesity, which is twice as prevalent in people who watch 3 to 4 hours of television per day.[24] With obesity often comes elevated blood fats, which results in sluggish immune function. The fact that couch potatoes exercise less should also not be overlooked. When you're on the couch, you're not out and about. Moderate exercise improves resistance to virtually all diseases.

Exercise: Good Preventive for Most Ailments

Exercise stimulates circulation, improves muscle tone, improves cardiac function and boosts immunity. It is also a way to eliminate toxins from the body. In Chapter 5 we discussed the myriad toxins that build up in the body as a result of regular bodily processes, in addition to exposure to man-made chemicals. Exercise is a critical component in the elimination of these "poisons" from the body for three simple reasons. First, when we exercise we breathe more deeply, more forcefully and more often. In doing so, we release toxic by-products through the lungs. Second, when we exercise we also perspire. Perspiration is another means to eliminate metabolic waste material from the body. Finally, muscular activity is *the only way* to move waste material through the lymphatic vessels. If we don't sweat, don't breathe heavily and don't move our muscles, these toxins must find another way out. Unfortunately, they usually remain in the body, only to foul the biochemical machinery that makes our immune system operate efficiently. The result: susceptibility to illness.

An article published in the *International Journal of Sports Medicine* illustrates the effect exercise can have on infections. In this study, only 45 minutes of brisk walking per day was shown to lower the incidence of upper respiratory symptoms, cut the duration of illness in half and increase natural killer-cell activity in people prone to upper respiratory tract infections.[25]

The exercise credo of the eighties, "no pain, no gain," has fortunately given way to a more realistic notion that moderate exercise confers as many health benefits as strenuous exercise. Moderate exercisers have the added benefit of suffering fewer injuries. So don't feel you have to pump iron with Schwarzenegger, sprint with Carl Lewis or cycle the Alps with Greg LeMond to get in shape. In fact, highly strenuous training can temporarily weaken immune function. When researchers at Loma Linda University studied runners of the Los Angeles Marathon, they found immune function to be depressed for several hours. According to Dr. David Nieman, "Those who train more than 60 miles a week double their odds of getting sick, compared with a runner training less than 20 miles a week."[26]

Runners of the 1982 Marathon in Cape Town, South Africa, had twice the incidence of upper respiratory infections in the two weeks following the race of non-runners. Runners with the fastest times suffered from more infections than runners with slower times.[27] Whether these effects are due to the act of running, the stress of anticipating a big race or both, no one is sure. However, if you are a heavy trainer who suffers from frequent infections, you may do well to consider decreasing the intensity of your training schedule.

While intensive training, or "pushing it to the wall" is what some prefer, rest assured that dancing, hiking, golfing (if you walk), walking, cross country skiing, swimming, volleyball, bicycling, bowling, shoveling snow, chopping wood and even sex provide your body with health and immune benefits. The key: make sure you exercise regularly and moderately, and make sure it's fun! (If you have an existing medical condition, see your doctor before embarking on any exercise plan.)

The Power of Prayer

Saying "grace" or giving thanks before a meal has been a component of many spiritual traditions for centuries. It is a display of gratitude to the Creator who has provided for basic needs. Recently, scientists have begun to study the effects of prayer on the body with some interesting results. In one study, investigators wondered whether prayer had any impact on digestive efficiency as measured by after-meal comfort. Subjects were asked to rate the feeling in their "tummy"on a scale of 1 to 10, 1 being poor and 10 being excellent. They then sat down and consumed a meal and rated their feeling. The average was about 3. In the next test, each member said a silent prayer—the number rose to 4. On another day, they had one person in the group say a prayer of thanks aloud—the average score increased again. Then, each group member prayed aloud in unison with the others—the score rose further. Finally, all members held hands and prayed aloud together—the score rose to 8.[28] Do the results of this subjective test mean prayer improves digestion or anything else? Is it the prayer itself or the state of mind and body that occurs with the introspection brought about by prayer? It is hard to draw conclusions, but this study suggests that, if nothing else, the meditative state of active prayer may enhance digestive activity.

This raises the equally intriguing question of whether praying for another person has any real merit. Religions throughout the ages have believed the power of prayer to be boundless, unaffected by time or distance. Cardiologist Randy Byrd, a former professor of medicine at the University of California, attempted to answer the question of whether prayer influenced recovery from illness by enrolling 393 coronary care patients in a landmark study. One hundred ninety-two patients were to be prayed for each day by anonymous participants. The prayers were specific, including the name of the patient, their condition and a request that there be "beneficial healing and quick recovery." The 201 remaining coronary patients received no prayer. Patients were unaware they were being prayed for. This study was conducted under the most stringent scientific guidelines.

During the next 10 months, Dr. Byrd's research team followed these patients and analyzed the data. The subjects receiving prayer suffered significantly fewer complications than the control group. Remarkably, the prayed-for patients were *five times less likely to require antibiotics* than those who received no prayer.[29]

Another group of researchers showed that prayer had a dramatic effect on the growth of plants, especially when the plants were unhealthy. Again, these studies were conducted under the most rigorous double-blind, placebo-controlled conditions.[30]

Prayer does not guarantee that one will not become ill. Indeed, those who pray suffer from the same maladies as those who do not. Yet, prayer has the potential to move us beyond our limited perceptions of the world and of illness. In the next chapter we speak of illness as metaphor. Prayer and meditation may help give us insight into the greater meaning of periods of illness (assuming there is greater meaning to such periods).

Drugs and Alcohol

Earlier in this chapter, we discussed the adverse effects of smoking and how it suppresses the immune system. The same is true for drugs (both *legal* and *illegal)* and alcohol. Whether these substances come from the chemistry tubes of a pharmaceutical company, the vats of a distillery or winery, or the slopes of Colombian hillsides, the end result is the same: *Toxic Overload.*

Humans do not have ethanol or cocaine or Prozac or nicotine "deficiencies." They use these recreationally or medically, then gradually suffer the ill effects as their body tries its best to detoxify these foreign substances. When they are detoxified, they are excreted in the urine, the stool, sweat or in our breath as we exhale. If not excreted in these ways, these complex chemicals/poisons are stored in the liver, body fat or somewhere in the lymph nodes or other parts of the lymphatic system. When this overload exceeds the body's ability to function, illness follows.

AIDS is often cited as an example of how the immune system is impacted by drugs. Many of the first people who contracted AIDS had abused alcohol, nicotine, marijuana, cocaine or other drugs for years prior to the invasion of the HIV virus. They often led single, lonely and stressful lives. Their nutritional status was often suboptimal. Many had suffered from depression and were treated with antidepressants. Antibiotics were commonly overused, especially in homosexuals to treat sexually transmitted diseases. In many such cases, their immune systems were "wobbly." Often, they simply shut down. Such people were commonly sick *before* they got AIDS.

Lack of Sleep

Shakespeare wrote that sleep is the "chief restorer of life's feast." In modern terms that would mean that nearly one-third of Americans are "underfed." Because of that, they are irritable, moody, and unable to concentrate on their work and make mistakes in everyday tasks.

James Walsh, director of the Sleep Disorders and Research Center at Deaconess Hospital in St. Louis, attributes the 1984 Bhopal gas leak and the Exxon *Valdez* oil spill in part to misjudgements by sleep-deprived workers. The U.S. Department of Transportation estimates that drowsy drivers contribute to as many as 200,000 automobile accidents each year.

We all have different sleep needs. Leonardo da Vinci is said to have slept only two hours a day. Others need up to eight or ten hours of sleep to function at their best. According to the Institute of Medicine, an estimated 29 to 39 percent of Americans over the age of 18 have significant difficulty sleeping each year.[31] Failure to get adequate sleep leads to fatigue, which can impair our resistance to illness and our ability to cope with stressful events. Noted British physician James Paget once wrote, "Fatigue has a larger share in the promotion and transmission of disease than any other single condition you can name."[32]

Dr. J. M. Krueger reports that the onset of slow-wave sleep correlates with a surge in the blood levels of chemicals that stimulate immune function.[33] Lack of sleep is associated with increased susceptibility to stress and infections.

Rules for Better Sleep Hygiene[34]

1. Sleep as much as needed to feel refreshed and healthy during the following day, but not more. Curtailing the time in bed seems to solidify sleep; excessively long times in bed seem related to fragmented and shallow sleep.

2. A regular arousal time in the morning strengthens circadian cycling, and finally, leads to regular times of sleep onset.

3. A steady daily amount of exercise probably deepens sleep; occasional exercise does not necessarily improve sleep the following night.

4. Occasional loud noises (e.g. aircraft flyovers) disturb sleep even in people who are not awakened by noises and cannot remember them in the morning. Sound-attenuated bedrooms may help those who must sleep close to noise.

5. Although excessively warm rooms disturb sleep, there is no evidence that an excessively cold room solidifies sleep.

6. Hunger may disturb sleep; a light snack may help sleep.

7. An occasional sleeping pill may be of some benefit, but their chronic use is ineffective in most insomniacs. [Valerian root is an effective alternative to sleeping pills.]

8. Caffeine in the evening disturbs sleep, even in those who feel it does not.

9. Alcohol helps tense people fall asleep more easily, but the ensuing sleep is fragmented.

10. People who feel angry and frustrated because they cannot sleep should not try harder and harder to fall asleep but should turn on the light and do something different.

11. The chronic use of tobacco disturbs sleep.

The Search for Meaningful Touch

The skin is the largest sense organ in the body. Stimulation of the skin of the entire body is an important component of maintaining healthy contact with our external world and fostering health in our internal world. Unfortunately, many of us have become touch-starved.

When premature babies were massaged three times per day, they gained 28 percent more weight over a 10-day period than did babies who were not massaged. They were also less easily startled and smiled more often. In a study at Duke University, researchers showed that massage increased levels of certain digestive hormones, allowing babies to more efficiently absorb nutrients from their food. Massage also lowers anxiety in children.[35]

Appropriate touch benefits growth, development and immune function. In a series of animal experiments, those given frequent touch utilized food better, developed more rapidly, learned more efficiently and showed greater emotional stability in stressful situations. Remarkably, *when confronted with stressful stimuli, the output of stress hormones was considerably lower in animals that received frequent touch than in those receiving less touch.*[36]

When animals are touched or handled extensively in infancy they show, as adults, more efficiently developed immune systems than animals that have received less tactile stimulation. They suffer fewer infections and have a lower mortality rate than their lesser-touched counterparts.[37]

In subtle, but profound ways, touch even influences our perception of people and events. Robert Tisserand reports on a study conducted at Purdue University in 1986. As students left the library after checking out books, they were asked questions regarding their opinion of the library and whether the librarian smiled at them. The library assistant treated everyone the same way, except that every other student was lightly touched on the hand as their library card was handed back to them. Those who were touched formed a more positive view of the library than those who were not and often thought that the assistant had smiled at them, even though she had not.[38]

Could you enhance immunity by more frequently touching your spouse and your children? Could you enhance your resistance to disease by getting a periodic massage? The evidence suggests that touch influences multiple aspects of human function and perception. Immunity is definitely among them.

Noise Pollution: A Twentieth-Century Creation

Noise pollution is a growing problem in our world of machinery and gadgets. Unwanted noise can create stress and contribute to a variety of physiological ills. Noise pollution can cause these problems alone, but it is more apt to cause problems if you perceive to have little or no control over the source of the noise or the noise level.

In Chapter 7, we discuss the impact of emotions, perception, coping and stress on immune function. Noise can have an insidious effect upon how we interpret and respond to events around us. For example, in a report published in *Psychology Today*, a researcher with a cast on one arm carried an armload of books and papers down the sidewalk and dropped them as another pedestrian approached. The researcher would then helplessly attempt to gather up the books. Nearby, another researcher was operating a power lawn mower. When the lawn mower was on, only 15 percent of the passers-by stopped to help pick up the books. In contrast, when the mower was silent, 80 percent stopped to lend a hand.[39]

According to Glenda Ochsner, professor at the University of Oklahoma Health Science Center, you can keep noise to a minimum by:[40]

- Using wallcoverings—fabric is best.
- Hang paintings or other art to break up a flat surface, which can bounce back sound.
- Use plants and furniture, both of which reduce echoing.
- Use rugs or carpets on floors.
- Place pads under countertop appliances.
- Designate a quiet place—a room in the house where people can relax without unwanted background noise.

Crowding

Crowding has historically been shown to contribute to the development and spread of infections. Animals who rarely succumb to infections in the wild succumb when confined in zoos. A classic example is the spread of infections in day care. Place a large number of children together in a crowded setting and a common outcome is the spread of parasites, coughs, colds, pneumonia, diarrheal illness and other common childhood disorders.

There has been a gradual trend toward urbanization in the West—more people are moving from the country to the city. Some believe that as this continues there will be a gradual increase in infectious illness. Air pollution, traffic, stress and crowding may act in concert to tax our immune systems.

Relaxation: The Immune Booster

When relaxation crept onto the medical scene, it was met with great skepticism. Gradually, it was shown that relaxation helped those with heart disease, cancer, diabetes and a variety of physical ills. Researchers then began to ask whether relaxation might cause an overall boost in immune function. The answer appears to be "yes." Today, hospitals and clinics all over the world are prescribing relaxation or meditation to patients for many different conditions.

But one need not be seriously ill to engage in meditation or relaxation. When practiced as a part of the daily routine, meditation can improve health at almost every level. According to Janice Kiecolt-Glaser, a researcher at Ohio State University, ". . . relaxation may be able to enhance some component of cellular immunity, and thus perhaps ultimately might be useful in influencing the incidence and course of disease."[41] In our clinical experience, patients who have learned to meditate and relax indeed seem to be healthier and more resistant to illness.

Are Doctors' Children the Healthiest?

The true test of the value of any health-promotion strategy is whether it actually works in real life. We (the authors) have proposed that by adopting practices of balance and holism in the way one lives, it is possible to prevent much illness and avoid antibiotics when one becomes ill with what appears to be an infection. One way to evaluate the effectiveness of such an approach is to study the families of groups of people who live by different philosophical beliefs and lifestyle practices.

The children of medical (allopathic) doctors would be a great bunch to study because they would theoretically have access to the "best" care available. Comparing the families of doctors who operated under different medical philosophies would be even better. Such a study was carried out by Drs. Wendy and Juan van Breda. The two researchers surveyed 200 pediatricians and 200 chiropractic physicians regarding the health status of their children. One can say in general that chiropractic physicians are more inclined to use nutrition, dietary therapy, homeopathy, herbs, acupuncture and spinal manipulation than their medical colleagues in pediatrics. Chiropractic physicians are likewise less inclined to resort to antibiotics when illness strikes. The findings of the researchers were striking. Nearly 50 percent of the children of chiropractors had never received antibiotics. This was in sharp contrast to that of the pediatricians' children in whom less than 12 percent had not used these drugs.

Were the chiropractors' children more healthy? Or did the fact that they had not taken antibiotics suggest they were receiving inferior care? According to the researchers, 69 percent of the chiropractic children reported *no occurrence* of middle ear infection and 73 percent reported no tonsillitis. Of the children raised under allopathic care, only 20 percent reported no ear infections while 57 percent reported no tonsillitis. The researchers offered this conclusion. They wrote, "This study has shown that children raised under chiropractic care are less prone to infectious processes such as otitis media and tonsillitis, and that their immune systems are better able to cope with allergens such as pollens, weeds, grasses, etc., as compared to children raised under allopathic [medical] care."[42]

While one could choose to argue with the conclusion of the researchers, the findings at least deserve serious consideration. At best, they suggest a breakthrough in the prevention and treatment of illness in children. If a study came out showing that a *new drug* could reduce our reliance on antibiotics by 40 percent or that we could dramatically reduce the incidence of ear infections, tonsillitis, allergy and asthma, it would be heralded as one of the greatest medical discoveries of this quarter century. Yet the above survey does not deal with a drug and has received scant attention.

The National Institutes of Health (NIH) should be busy studying the families who have reduced their rate of illness (in comparison to the population at-large) and who have reduced their reliance on antibiotics. Given the problems with antibiotics outlined in Chapter 2, it seems only logical. Unfortunately, the NIH is not likely to do so. However, one doesn't need the NIH to show the way. By adopting a strategy of balance and holism in your life you can optimize wellness. You also have freedom to choose the doctor of your choice.

Healthy Pleasures

Doctors tend to be risk managers. Usually that means they tell you what to avoid in order to stay healthy. Indeed, this book is filled with some of the same admonitions. But a question always arises over why some people, despite horrible dietary habits, coffee consumption, late-night voyeurism, and altogether decadent lifestyles seem to "get off" with little or no illness, while one who works hard, eats right, sleeps well and takes vitamins is beset with health problems. Chapter 7 may hold some of the answers because attitude and emotional make-up play an important role. Yet there is more. Is it possible that "going for the gusto," taking pleasure in all of life's moments, exploring some of the "no-nos," is the key to well-being? Is it possible that laughing at the world's travails as well as your own foibles, while ignoring the dogged realism of life promotes health? Could it be that chocolate is the way to happiness?

Robert Ornstein, Ph.D., and David Sobel, M.D., might argue that the answer is "yes." In their book *Healthy Pleasures,* they write, "Many people today are concerned about living longer, feeling better, and having more energy, so there is a continuing demand for good health advice. Still, something is missing from all these recommendations, be they about nutrition, exercise, surgery, drug therapy, meditation, or stress relief: the vital role of pleasure. *Healthy Pleasures* proposes a new approach to the way women and men manage their health. We believe that it can be done better with less effort and with much more fun."

They state that "the healthiest people seem to be pleasure-loving, pleasure-seeking, pleasure-creating individuals." So, while we share many ideas that help promote wellness, be aware that rigid determinism and suffering for the cause of good health is not likely to bear fruit. The search for optimum health can be enjoyable.[43]

A Summary of Things to Do

In this chapter we have discussed just a few of the important factors that influence our resistance to infection. There are certainly many more. We believe that by adopting some basic changes in lifestyle, one can enhance immunity. A summary of helpful things is below.

1. Get moderate exercise on a regular basis. Make sure it is interesting and enjoyable.

2. Don't smoke or use chewing tobacco.

3. Avoid excessive TV viewing. If you watch TV, get up and turn down the sound whenever a commercial appears. It will prevent you from stagnating on the couch and free you from advertisements for high-sugar, high-fat junk food.

4. Pray or meditate each day.

5. Look at the health of your parents and siblings. If they are prone to certain types of illness, you may be likewise. Take preventive steps regarding lifestyle and nutrition.

6. Drink alcohol only moderately, if at all.

7. Avoid overuse of prescription drugs.

8. Avoid use of illicit drugs.

9. Get plenty of sunlight, especially in winter months. In the summer, avoid excessive sunlight. Balance is the key.

10. Take a weekly sauna, especially in winter months. First check with your doctor if you are pregnant or have cardiovascular or other medical problems.

11. Get adequate sleep. Most people need 6 to 8 hours a night of uninterrupted sleep. A short nap in the afternoon is often helpful, provided it does not disrupt your evening sleep.

12. Limit the amount of noise present in your home and workplace. If you cannot limit the source of the noise, take steps to limit its effect on you.

13. Bring more touch into your life. Consider getting a periodic massage from a professional massage therapist.

14. Have fun. Seek pleasure and meaning in all you do.

7

Mood, Mind, Stress and Infections

"Our susceptibility to infectious disease . . . has now been convincingly linked to the way we cope with our life and environment."
Blair Justice, Ph.D.
Who Gets Sick[1]

In 1991, an article appeared in the journal *Stress Research* estimating that 60 percent of all visits to family doctors are prompted by emotionally induced, stress-related symptoms. According to Bernice C. Sachs, M.D., "Stress has probably now surpassed the common cold as the most prevalent health problem in America."[2] Workers' compensation claims related to stress tripled during the first half of the 1980s. Today, of disability claims by professionals, the vast majority are stress-related. The fact that the top-selling prescription drugs in the United States are those used for nervous disorders and depression further suggests that stress and emotional factors are among the major health problems in this country.

There are many definitions of stress. Psychiatrist Stephen Locke describes stress as "the perception of individuals that their life circumstances have exceeded their capacity to cope."[3] Noted personality researcher H. J. Eysenck points out that we must distinguish between "stress" and "strain" much as an engineer or a physicist would. Stress is the outside force brought to bear upon the individual. Strain is our reaction to the outside force.[4] Dr. Hans Selye, who is credited with bringing the concept of stress to public atten-

155

tion, gave this definition: "Stress is the nonspecific response of the body to any demand made upon it."[5] Selye realized that some stress was necessary for survival. He made a distinction between pleasurable or 'eustress' and painful or 'dis-stress.'

During the past two decades, scientists have learned that stress can have a profound effect on immune function and susceptibility to disorders ranging from infectious disease to arthritis to cancer.

Stress, Life Events & Infections

Infectious disease expert Dr. Tohru Ishegami observed at the turn of the century that the principal factor determining whether tuberculosis patients would survive or succumb to this infectious disease was their emotional state. He realized that stressful life events took a toll on patients suffering from tuberculosis (TB). Stress seemed to be predictive of who became sick and who did not become sick. It also seemed to explain why reasonably healthy individuals became seriously ill. Dr. Ishegami commented on the factors that influence susceptibility to TB. He stated, "The personal history usually reveals failure in business, lack of harmony in the family, or jealousy of some sort. Nervous individuals are especially prone to attacks of this type, and the prognosis is generally bad." He continued, "Again, in chronic cases, patients may go on apparently well until some misfortune happens. This immediately alters the course of the disease."[6]

This "novel" concept that stress and life events might influence the course of infectious disease was published in 1919. Since Dr. Ishegami's time, the germ theory of disease and antibiotic treatments dominated the medical scene. Little attention was given to the psychosocial aspects of infection. Only since about 1980 have we seen the emergence of a concerted effort to understand infection from this perspective.

Dr. W. Thomas Boyce and his colleagues raised several important questions regarding infections in children. They wrote, "Despite major advances in the microbiology of respiratory disease, why and how a child becomes ill remain poorly understood. In over half of respiratory illnesses, complete cultures fail to yield an etiologic [infectious or causative] agent. Conversely, 30 percent of a school-age population can harbor group A *Streptococci* without developing symptoms, three-quarters of preschool children infected with *Mycoplasma pneumoniae* remain asymptomatic, and as many as 42 percent of upper respiratory tract cultures from well children yield pneumococci."[7]

Dr. Boyce and his colleagues at the University of North Carolina-Chapel Hill believed that stressful events in the life of children played a role in why some children became sick while others exposed to the same infectious germs did not. They also theorized that having well-established routines such as waking, bathing, eating, napping and playing at the same time each day would be protective against the adversity of stressful events.

They sought to test their hypothesis through a carefully designed study. Each child was scored on a "Life Events" test that looked at the relative degree of stress brought about by difficult life changes such as death of a grandparent, parental divorce, a move to a new city and so on. (These were based on the original work by Holmes and Rahe, who developed the Social Readjustment Rating Scale.) Each child was then observed daily for signs of respiratory illness. In addition, nasopharyngeal cultures were taken to determine whether viruses or bacteria were present.

After factoring out all variables such as age, sex, race, income and family size, the researchers found that "life change scores were significantly and independently predictive of the average *duration* of illness." Then a surprising finding emerged. High life change (or life event) scores *coupled with* rigid family routines were together related to the *severity* of illness. According to Boyce, "It appears that illnesses became more severe as the magnitude of life change and the strength of family routines jointly increased." Dr. Boyce was surprised to find that routine helped to increase rather than decrease susceptibility to severe illness. The researchers concluded that:

- Life change was the strongest single predictor of how long a child stayed ill.
- Major life change in the setting of a highly ritualized family appeared to predispose to greater illness severity.
- Scores for life change and family routines had no noticeable influence on the growth of harmful bacteria or

viruses from the respiratory tract in either health or
disease.

While life changes and routine affected duration and severity of
illness, they did not affect the presence of germs in the respiratory
tract. In other words, bacteria and viruses were present in both
high-stress and low-stress children, but the high-stress children suffered from more prolonged and severe illness.

This finding is similar to that of an earlier study in which 16
families were followed for one year. Every three weeks each family member had a physical exam that included a throat culture for
streptococcal bacteria. Family members also kept diaries docu-
menting events that occurred during the one-year test period.

At the end of one year, researchers reviewed the data to determine whether there was an association between stressful life events
and illness. They discovered that:

- Stress was four times more likely to precede an infection
  as to follow an infection.

- When throat cultures revealed a streptococcal infection,
  one-half of those under high stress became ill.

- Of the low-stress individuals with a positive strep. culture,
  only *one-fifth* became ill.

- One out of four outbreaks of illness followed some form
  of family crisis.[8]

No one has gone so far as to say stress causes infections. But
as the above studies show, stress and life events indeed have a significant impact on susceptibility to infection. Dr. Hans Selye offered
this observation in 1978. He wrote, "If a microbe is in or around us
all the time and yet causes no disease until we are exposed to stress,
what is the 'cause' of our illness, the microbe or the stress? I think
both are and equally so. In most instances the disease is due . . .
to the inadequacy of our reactions against the germ."[9]

This raises the important question, "how appropriate are antibiotics when stressful events might be at the root of infection susceptibility?" Are doctors acting inappropriately when they prescribe
antibiotics without understanding the context in which infections
occur?

Mood, Mind, Stress and Infections

Consider the following case. David was a 35-year-old accountant with a wife, two small children and another child on the way. He was unhappy in his job, had recently moved to a new home, but was unable to sell his previous home. After nearly one year of paying for two homes, he found a party interested in buying his home. Then, just as they were getting ready to sell, a week of torrential rains caused the basement to flood. The FHA agent in charge of the sale decided that many costly improvements (to prevent further flooding) had to be made in order to grant the loan. On several successive occasions, the deal was to close, only to have the FHA agent demand another round of compliance. With each new edict, Dave became further enraged, further out of control. Meanwhile, his pregnant wife had fallen down the stairs and began contractions. They thought the baby was injured and coming prematurely. Fortunately, mother and child were OK.

After several thousand dollars in additional expenses, months of extra work and weeks off his job, the closing date finally arrived. The night before closing, the agent called Dave to say his buyers would no longer pay the "points"—he would have to pay. Dave was ready to take the whole matter to court, but then relented. The deal closed, Dave went home, crashed into bed and woke up hours later with a high fever, flaming red swollen tonsils, delirium and chills. Dave's immune system was "rattled" by stress. He reached the breaking point and succumbed to an opportunistic "germ" that might not have otherwise affected him.

The imbalance with which our current medical system addresses the issue of infection—favoring the germ theory and antibiotic therapy—can be further illustrated by a research project conducted by Donald M. Cassata, Ph.D., while on staff at the University of Minnesota. Cassata described a case in which a father entered a medical clinic with his young daughter who was suffering from recurrent ear infections. The resident doctor entered the examination room and immediately questioned the father about his daughter's complaint. The doctor examined the ears, listened to her lungs, checked her eyes and nasal passages and performed a general physical exam. The physician concluded that the girl was suffering from upper respiratory congestion and otitis media (middle ear inflammation). He then pulled out his prescription pad and wrote a prescription for four different drugs, one of which was an antibiotic. After writing the prescription, the doctor left the examination room.

One focus of this study was to evaluate the medical resident's performance. He received high marks from his professors who were observing via video hook-up. The resident asked the "right" questions, did the "right" exam, and prescribed the "right" drugs.

Then came Dr. Cassata, who thought it odd that a father had brought his daughter to the clinic rather than the mother. (At the time of this study, fathers were rarely seen bringing sick children to a clinic.) Dr. Cassata asked how the family was doing. The father broke into tears as he described the tragic battle his wife had waged with cancer. He described the toll his wife's illness had taken on the family. His young daughter had taken her mother's illness especially hard, becoming ill with recurrent earaches not long after her mother learned of her cancer.[10]

Loss of a family member, threat of loss of a family member and prolonged illness of a parent are always listed among events producing the greatest degree of stress in both children and adults. Bereavement has been repeatedly shown to produce deficiencies in immune function.

From the previous studies, it is clear that bacteria and viruses do not necessarily cause disease. A combination of the infectious organism and lowered resistance to infection may be required in order for one to become ill from infection. In this girl's case, was antibiotic treatment appropriate? It may have been. Then again, in the absence of dealing with the family dynamics and the loss of the girl's mother, antibiotic therapy may have been wholly inappropriate. Since antibiotics do nothing to enhance immune function, they would likely not improve her resistance to infection. This girl may well have mounted the tragic treadmill of repeated antibiotics and recurrent infections.

Stress and the Common Cold

The most universal affliction of humans—the common cold—also appears to be influenced by stress. When individuals were exposed to one of five common cold viruses, 90 percent of those under high stress became infected compared with only 74 percent of those under low stress. Of those in the low-stress group, only 27 percent actually became ill. This was in contrast to 47 percent of those in the high stress group suggesting that stress nearly doubles the likelihood of becoming ill when exposed to a cold virus.[11]

Dr. Sheldon Cohen and his associates in the Department of Psychology at Carnegie Mellon University observed that the stress-infection connection occurred among three very different viruses (rhinovirus, coronavirus and respiratory syncytial virus), leading them to conclude ". . . stress is associated with the suppression of a general resistance process in the host, leaving persons susceptible to multiple infectious agents . . . stress is associated with the suppression of many different immune processes, with similar results."[12]

Black Monday Syndrome

Perhaps nothing illustrates the mortal effects of stress better than what has come to be called "Black Monday Syndrome." More fatal heart attacks occur between 8 and 9 A.M. Monday morning than at any other time or day of the week. This was a startling finding to many doctors, but has since been confirmed by at least fourteen studies. Researchers have suggested that the stress of returning to a job one dreads causes the release of chemicals within the body that can trigger a heart attack in someone at risk. The larger meaning here is that job stress can have significant physiological effects. The ones who die are the ones we hear about. According to Larry Dossey, M.D., of the Dallas Diagnostic Association, humans are the only species on the planet that die more frequently on one day of the week.[13]

Stress and the Immune System

It was not long ago that doctors believed the immune system operated completely independent of all other body systems. As research began to support a link between mind and immunity, however, it became evident that thoughts, feelings and images have a direct impact upon immune function. But how?

Many researchers were stunned with the discovery that the immune system is "hard wired" to the nervous system. Nerve fibers of the autonomic nervous system—our automatic pilot—branch directly into the tissue of the lymph nodes, spleen, bone marrow and thymus gland. They are in *direct communication* with pools of white blood cells. Moreover, white blood cells have been shown to possess receptors on their surfaces for neurochemicals such as adrenaline and noradrenaline.

Scientists once believed that these neurochemicals acted *only* on nerves. They were the messengers that carried information from nerve cell to nerve cell. With the remarkable finding of a direct neurochemical link between the nervous and immune systems came implications for our understanding of health and disease. Mind and immunity are connected. The brain and immune system are engaged in a constant dialogue. The immune system increasingly seems to act like a "wandering nervous system" that is inextricably linked to our state of mind.

When the body is under stress, it releases chemicals that play a survival role. An ancient hunter startled by a charging tiger needed quick action to save himself. His body released adrenaline and cortisol, which provided an instant burst of strength and energy. He sped for cover—the "flight" phase of the "fight or flight" response.

An auto mechanic working under a car is trapped when the jack fails. His coworker, seeing the threat of death or injury to his partner, experiences a sudden surge of cortisol and adrenaline. In a display of near-superhuman strength, he lifts the car off his friend—the "fight" phase.

These brief threat and response situations can have adverse immune consequences. Fortunately, the effects of this type of stress are generally short-lived and produce little difficulty.

When stress is prolonged, however, the release of stress hormones like cortisol continues. The bereaved spouse, the executive continually having to meet deadlines, the commuter mired in daily rush-hour traffic, mates embroiled in bitter divorce proceedings—all are faced with persistent and ongoing stress. They are in a constant "fight or flight" mode with no one to fight and nowhere to run! Prolonged elevation of cortisol can cause destruction of T-cells in the thymus gland and the release of T-cells before they mature. This combination leads to a gradual shrinking of the thymus, the master gland of the immune system.

The effect of stress on immune function is not thoroughly understood. We do know that the nervous and immune systems communicate in complex ways. Some compounds stimulate immune function while others suppress it. Prolonged physical, psychological or social distress decreases immune vigilance and increases susceptibility to disease by a variety of means. The most common stressors include:

1. Biological Stressors: Bacteria, viruses, parasites, yeast, mold and fungi.

2. Environmental Stressors: Noise, extremes of temperature, extremes of humidity, lack of sunlight, excess sunlight, air pollution, water pollution, traumatic accidents.

3. Emotional Stressors: Anger, hostility, cynicism, resentment, fear anxiety, hatred.

4. Deprivation Stressors: Lack of humor, laughter, joy, love, touch, fun, silliness, meaningful relationships, sleep, exercise . . .

5. Social Stressors: Crowding, world events, crime, racism, war.

6. Family Stressors: Divorce, marriage, separation, death, birth of child, changes in work status, abusive relationships, changes in financial status, college.

Usually, one of these factors alone is insufficient to alter our resistance to disease. However, when we accumulate stressors, our resistance gradually declines, rendering us more susceptible to a variety of ills, especially infections by organisms already present in our bodies and environment.

Negative Effects from Stress Are Not Inevitable

The discovery of a link between stress and immune function was one of the greatest discoveries of this century (although adherents to ancient traditions would rightly argue it was merely recognition and verification of what has been known for centuries). Yet, as this work progressed, a puzzling finding emerged. Some individuals, despite innumerable stressors and tragedy upon tragedy, seemed little affected. What were the "mysterious" qualities that allowed some to rise above the heavy hand dealt by fate and circumstance? What allowed them to persevere in the face of overwhelming odds? That story is unfolding today. It is clear that many human qualities are important determinants of whether we succumb to the ravages of stress or whether we "carry on." As Larry Dossey, M.D., states, "We should always recall that, no matter how stressful the event, we can always bring our attitudes, beliefs, and meanings to bear on the situation and change its effects on us."[14]

It's Not Always the Stress, But How We Cope

As we noted previously, stress is brought about by many different phenomena: social, personal, climatic, environmental, nutritional and so on. Someone once likened stress to a hurricane. It can whip through town and leave damage that might take years to repair. How one recovers from the damage and how quickly depends on many factors. Why some people are more vulnerable than others is something the experts still struggle with, but it seems to be linked to our perception of events and our ability to cope. Events that might be crippling for one individual might be seen as a challenge for another. Those that might trigger depression in one person may spur another to greater achievement. Why the difference?

While we recognize the importance of stress as a factor in illness, we emphasize that humans are not merely unwitting victims of life's events. Given adequate coping skills, social support, attitude or whatever the key, you can overcome the effects of stress in your life. Though some of the darts of stress may stick, you can become more efficient at deflecting the bulk of those that come your way.

The ability to cope with stressful events may be what sets those who rise above the forces of stress apart from those who succumb to them. Coping skills can be learned, but there may be aspects of your personality *coupled with* the environment in which you find yourself that affect how you cope. For instance, managers who are of the Type-A personality (competitive, driven, overly time-conscious) prefer a working environment that allows them a great degree of autonomy and individuality. When working in an environment that encourages independence, these individuals are less stressed and at less risk to illness from stress. Put this person in a highly structured environment where someone else calls all the shots, and their blood pressure skyrockets.

In contrast, Type-B people who are more laid-back, less time-urgent and generally less competitive* prefer structure. When working in an environment that requires independence and autonomy, these people become more stressed and suffer higher blood pressure. The Type-B person is often more comfortable and copes better in a more structured environment.[15]

Perception and Control

One's coping skills are greatly affected by the *perception* of events. In fact, perception may be one of the most critical determinants of how people respond to stress. For example, in surveys of what people say they fear most, public speaking is always listed at the top (well ahead of fear of heights and even death). Someone unaccustomed to public speaking may begin to develop anxiety attacks months in advance of the speaking date. As the date approaches, the anxiety grows. Some individuals are so affected, they become ill. They perceive public speaking as a threatening experience. On the other hand, seasoned speakers look forward to speaking engagements as an opportunity to share their ideas, challenge the crowd and get feedback. To them, speaking in public is just part of their job or perhaps a means to advance a social cause. To them, speaking is exhilarating, not stressful.

For roughly 25 percent of the population, flying in an airplane is a stressful event. Some venture bravely onto airplanes simply because it is the only way to get where they want to go. Others avoid flying altogether. For the bulk of the population, however, flying is "no big deal." There is little stress involved other than airport hassles, flight delays and lost luggage.

---

*Type-B people are certainly competitive and succeed to the same degree as Type-A people. They are just not competitive to the extreme that Type-A people are competitive.

Consider the case of Bill and Beth. Beth was scheduled to have major surgery the day after Christmas. A uterine tumor had caused a number of chronic health complaints. Beth was eagerly awaiting removal of the tumor, anticipating that her health problems would soon be solved. Her chronic illness, the stress of the holidays and the impending surgery seemed a heavy burden—not to mention the fact that most of her family was out of town, unable to support her. However, her optimistic view of the likely outcome minimized the impact of these stressors. She went into surgery feeling reasonably well and recovered quite well.

Bill was a different story. It was Christmas and his wife was facing major surgery. He would have to care for her and their small children during the recovery period; he was not totally convinced the surgery was best; he was worried about what else the surgeons might find; and he was unfamiliar with surgical procedures. He had no control. On Christmas Eve Bill came down with the flu accompanied by two full days of nausea, vomiting and diarrhea. By the day of Beth's surgery, he had recovered sufficiently to go to the hospital with her and offer support.

You might imagine that Beth had more stress than her husband since she was to have surgery. Why then did Bill succumb to the flu (a common stress reaction) while Beth remained unaffected? Why did he appear to respond differently to stressful events that similarly faced Beth? There may be several reasons. Beth had an optimistic view of the outcome of her surgery. She *perceived* the surgery as an opportunity to improve her health. Moreover, Beth had more *control*—Bill had little. Control, real or perceived, is a critical element in how we manage stress. It affects whether we succumb to the forces of stress or whether we rise above them.

A remarkable study was performed to illustrate how profoundly control affects us. Two groups of people were exposed to a very annoying and stress-inducing noise. One group was exposed to the noise with no means to reduce or control it. The other group was told that if they pushed a button on the arm of their chair, the noise would be reduced. Subjects in the second group were unaware that the button had no effect whatsoever on the noise level. The stress response of the two groups was dramatically different. The group able to push the button, even though the button had no effect on the noise, suffered far fewer symptoms of stress than the other group. The reason: they believed they had control over their environment and the belief translated into real bodily changes.[16]

Perception of our own health status can have an equally dramatic effect on our well-being. Researchers posed the following question to 2,800 people over the age of 65, "At the present time, how would you rate your health: excellent, good, fair, poor or bad?" It was discovered that men who answered "excellent" were nearly seven times as likely to be alive four years later than men in apparently similar states of health who answered "poor" or "bad." Women who answered "excellent" were more than seven times as likely to be alive as similar women who answered "poor" or "bad." According to Dr. Ellen Idler, health and aging researcher at Rutgers University, similar studies comparing self-perception with the results of complete physical exams have led to similar findings in people of all ages.[17,18] These findings suggest, in essence, that even though two people might be similar in their "actual" physical health, one who perceives his health as excellent lives longer and is healthier, while one who perceives his health as "poor" or "bad" suffers more illness and dies sooner.

Power Coping and the Art of Letting Go

One of the most dramatic tools for coping with our lives is the ancient but simple act of confession. James W. Pennebaker, professor of psychology at Southern Methodist University (SMU) in Dallas, has made a career of studying the effect of confession on health. He has shown that those who share their deepest feelings about past or present trauma are better able to cope and are healthier than those who do not share such feelings.

The two most common means of confession are talking and writing. In a study at SMU, Pennebaker asked his freshmen students to write about their deepest anxieties and their feeling about the dramatic changes involved in beginning college. He calls this "power coping." Those students who wrote about their current anxieties had fewer illnesses and visits to the doctor over the next four months. Those who wrote about only trivial or superficial topics showed a gradual increase in visits to the doctor.

Pennebaker wondered if such a decrease in illness was due to an actual increase in immune vigilance. In another study he and his colleagues actually measured the activity of T-cells, important in protecting us from infectious disease. His group found that those who wrote about past trauma had an increase in T-cell activity. Subjects who wrote about trauma they had not previously shared with anyone had the most dramatic rise in T-cell activity. As expected, those who wrote about traumas also had a decrease in visits to the health center.

Pennebaker's findings suggest that confession is a most powerful means of promoting a healthy immune system and health in general. There are several important keys to remember. Positive as well as "negative" experiences or emotions can be stressful or traumatic. Great and small events or experiences can also be stressful. Writing or verbal confession can be a superbly valuable way of letting go during these times.

It is important that you write for at least three or four days to achieve any benefit. Writing about trivial topics is generally not helpful. Writing about feelings and emotions is an essential part of deriving value from confession. One need not write every day, but when times are difficult or you sense your health level declining, writing may be a boon to well-being. Pennebaker's work is discussed in his excellent book *Opening Up: The Healing Power of Confiding in Others* (Avon, 1991). (An interview with Dr. Pennebaker appears in *EastWest Natural Health* July/August, 1992.)

Are You An Optimist or A Pessimist? Your Cells Know

In his wonderful book *Who Gets Sick,* medical writer Blair Justice begins a section with the definition of a pessimist. He writes, "A pessimist is someone who, when confronted with two unpleasant alternatives, selects both."[19] Taking his definition a step further, you might say that an optimist is one who, when confronted with these alternatives chooses neither, diminishes their significance or finds the positive possibilities in each. *The American Heritage Dictionary* defines an optimist as one who usually expects a favorable outcome.

Optimism is increasingly being viewed as an important part of a healthy immune system, while pessimism appears to be associated with lowered immunity. In an oft-cited study, researchers at the University of Michigan studied the effects of optimism/pessimism on the health of Harvard University graduates who were first interviewed in 1946 and followed for 35 years. Subjects were asked about difficult experiences encountered in World War II. The accounts were classified as global ("It will ruin my whole life"), stable ("It will never go away"), or internal ("It was all my fault"). Those with negative or pessimistic interpretations of their experiences were found to be consistently sicker than their more optimistic peers.[20]

The leader of this study, Dr. Christopher Peterson, listed a number of reasons why pessimism may contribute to more frequent illness:

- Pessimism may be linked to poor problem-solving ability and therefore to serious problems—hence, vulnerability to illness.

- Pessimism may lead to social withdrawal, behavior also associated with illness.

- Pessimism-related helplessness may affect immune function.

There is also direct evidence that optimists enjoy better immune function than pessimists. In their book *Healthy Pleasures,* David Sobel, M.D., and Robert Ornstein, Ph.D., report that when the blood of optimists is compared with that of pessimists, the optimists have higher levels of T-helper cells in relation to T-suppressors. Recall that T-helper cells stimulate immune function while T-suppressors suppress immune function. A high "helper" to "suppressor" ratio is desirable since resistance to infection and other illness would be enhanced.[21]

Martin Seligman, Ph.D., is Director of Clinical Training in Psychology at the University of Pennsylvania and is the leading researcher in the study of the effects of optimism on immune function. His observations after decades of extensive research include the following:

- Pessimists make twice as many visits to the doctor as optimists.

- Pessimists have *twice* as many infectious diseases as optimists.

- Optimists have more active and more efficient immune systems.

- Pessimism often leads to depression, which causes a downturn in immune function.

- Major life changes can cause a decrease in immune function. In optimists the effects are less severe than in pessimists.

- Statistically, pessimists encounter more negative life events. The more bad life events we encounter, the more illness we will likely experience.

According to Seligman, "If your level of pessimism can deplete your immune system, it seems likely that pessimism can impair your physical health over your whole life span."[22]

This finding of enhanced immunity among optimists appears to have some historical precedent. Infectious disease expert Dr. Tohru Ishegami, observed at the turn of the century that the principal factor determining whether tuberculosis patients would survive or succumb to the disease was their emotional state. Even in some of the most severe cases, patients prevailed over their illness. Commenting on such cases, Dr. Ishegami remarked, "These patients are found to be optimistic and not easily worried."[23]

The "eternal optimist" is often chided by her peers for putting a happy face on sometimes not-so-happy circumstances; for always finding the silver lining in every cloud; for downplaying the negatives of a situation while accentuating the positives. Yet it is becoming evident that the optimist's view of the world may, in fact, be the healthy view.

We can be comforted by the fact that pessimism is not a fate to which any of us are destined. According to Dr. Seligman, pessimism can be unlearned and optimism learned. The tools necessary for embarking on the road to optimism are outlined in his book *Learned Optimism*. A healthy dose of optimism, while not a cure for disease, may begin to give your immune system a boost. An added benefit is that it may make life more enjoyable.

Great Expectations

It is healthy to succeed as students, athletes, musicians, parents, as human beings. To place high expectations on ourselves is natural and generally beneficial. However, when expectations take the form of demands or we fall far short of our expectations, the effect can be negative. Parents who place unusual demands or expect too much of their children may be setting the stage for lowered immune function; likewise with spouses and co-workers.

Research conducted at Yale University by Stanislav Kasl and his colleagues lends support to this view. They looked at the enrollment and medical records of West Point cadets. Contained in the record was information about family history and background, including personal and parental expectations. The investigators were particularly interested in laboratory tests for Epstein-Barr virus, the cause of infectious mononucleosis. They wondered why some cadets infected with the virus became ill while others seemed unaffected.

The answer appeared to lie in the psychosocial record. Kasl found that the cadets who became ill shared three common features: The fathers were described as "overachievers"; the cadets were strongly committed to a military career; the cadets were performing poorly academically. The combined effect of poor performance and high expectations seemed to increase the likelihood of succumbing to infection. Surprisingly, as academic rank went down, the severity of the infection went up.[24]

When our performance does not meet our expectations, it can affect our health. To cope we must either work harder to improve our performance or lower our expectations. In the above study, cadets who did one or the other did not become sick or had relatively short illnesses.

Abuse and Illness

The rising tide of physical and emotional abuse in society is a sad reality. We are only beginning to understand the many ways in which humans are affected by abuse. One adverse effect of abuse seems to be an increase in susceptibility to disease. Tamerra P. Moeller and Gloria A. Bachmann of the University of Medicine and Dentistry of New Jersey recently tried to assess the effects of childhood abuse on the rate of illness in women. Their findings showed that 53 percent of the women reported suffering one or more kinds of abuse as children (physical, emotional or sexual). The women reporting abuse were more likely to report symptoms such as fatigue, insomnia and headaches. They also reported more illness and required more hospitalization than did those not reporting a history of childhood abuse.[25]

Power and Self-Efficacy

One's susceptibility to infection can presumably be affected by the level of power they are given over their lives. Individuals who are constantly told "you won't be able to do that," or "you'll never amount to anything," or "you're no good," or similar admonitions will often feel that they have limited capability. This is often referred to as self-efficacy. When confronted with tasks that are challenging or unfamiliar, such persons come under extreme emotional stress. Fearful that they will not perform or will be reprimanded if they perform poorly, they withdraw. In one study, such persons with a low feeling of self-efficacy were found to produce increased levels of adrenal hormones when asked to perform a difficult task. The amount of stress hormone released was often dependent upon the person's *perceived* ability to perform the task.[26] As noted earlier, the stress hormones have an adverse effect upon immune function.

Social Support and Meaningful Relationships

The North American Indians, the Australian Aborigines, the tribes of the Kalahari and countless other groups have throughout history relied on a close-knit social structure for survival. The social groups were important for gathering food and for protection. But there was more to the social group than fulfillment of physical needs. Close social networks provided stability and support for every group member during good times as well as during times of pain and deprivation. Following the death of a loved one, grieving tribal members were supported by the group. During illness, the sick were cared for not only by the healer (or shaman), but by parents, grandparents and other tribal members. During childbirth, mothers were supported by the "wise women" of the tribal group. This social support network provided the greatest insurance for survival of individuals and the group as a whole.

In today's individualistic and fast-paced world, the social network is eroding. We often sit idly in our living rooms with the VCR playing old movies. We work in communities far from those in which we live. We live thousands of miles from our parents and grandparents. Far too often we are not members of churches, synagogues or faith communities that were an integral part of our parent's traditions. The sense of community or belonging is critical to our well-being, but is sorely lacking today.

Having stable social ties apparently helps us resist disease even when known risk factors to disease are present. In the Surgeon General's report on smoking released in 1975, it was shown that there were 1,560 deaths per 100,000 people in those who smoked 20+ cigarettes per day. There were only 762 deaths for non-smokers. After careful analysis of the data, biophysicist Harold Moskowitz made a startling discovery. Divorced *non-smokers* suffered nearly the same death rate (1,420) as did married smokers. In smokers who were divorced, the death rate climbed to 2,675.[27] What was it about marriage that seemed to be protective?

For many years we've known that the Japanese have lower rates of heart disease than Americans. It was shown decades ago that Japanese moving to the United States developed heart disease at roughly the same rate as their American counterparts. This has been attributed primarily to differences in dietary habits between Americans and Japanese and has been supported by much research. However, recent studies of the Japanese provide a surprising twist. Japanese men who emigrated to the United States, *but retained strong social ties and links to Japanese culture,* suffered from far lower rates of heart disease than their Japanese cohorts who did not retain such ties. This was despite a relatively high-fat diet, high serum cholesterol, high blood pressure, cigarette smoking and alcohol consumption among many of the Japanese emigrés.[28]

While strong social ties and a close-knit support network appear to protect us from illness, there are obvious risks as well. According to Robert Ornstein, Ph.D., and David Sobel, M.D., ". . . social support is not a cure-all. Maintaining one's health is not as simple as four hugs a day or to smile and say 'have a nice day' to everyone. In fact, relationships can have their negative side. The more family members or close friends one has, the more vulnerable one is to experience the loss of a loved one. Relationships can be financially and emotionally draining; just ask the spouse of an alcoholic or children caring for invalid parents."[29]

Even so, humans are by nature social creatures. We need interaction and support from an inner circle of people who share our ideals and with whom we can bond. We need a feeling of connectedness to other people and to our environment.

Anger, Cynicism and Hostility

According to Dr. Redford Williams, a researcher in behavioral medicine at Duke University Medical Center, "Our studies indicate that hostile, suspicious anger is right up there with any other health hazard we know about." It seems that the risk to disease from anger is on a par with the risk posed by smoking, obesity and high fat diets.[30]

Dr. Mara Julius, an epidemiologist at the University of Michigan, designed a study to assess the effects of anger on women over an 18-year period. Each woman was asked to complete a questionnaire that helped pinpoint signs of long-term, suppressed anger. Dr. Julius found that women who scored high on the anger profile "were three times more likely to have died during the study than women who did not harbor such hostile feelings."[31]

While many studies now point to the ability of anger and hostility to contribute to early death, heart disease and other problems, no one has yet shown a link to infection susceptibility.

However, the work of Dr. Paul Ekman, a psychologist at the University of California at San Francisco, has shed some interesting light on the response of the body to different states of mind. Ekman found that anger caused heart beat and skin temperature to rise significantly. He also discovered that simply mimicking the facial expressions of anger produced the same response. Others have shown that visualizing oneself angry also produces dramatic changes in pulse, blood pressure and other physiologic functions.

Anger and hostility eat away at the substance of the human psyche. These emotions foster an atmosphere of negativity that clouds every human endeavor. Researchers are increasingly showing a link between anger, hostility and cynicism and the development of disease and premature death.

Redford Williams offers the following suggestions for curbing cynicism and hostility:[32]

1. Monitor your cynical thoughts. Keep a log of situations in which you respond cynically and attempt to evaluate them from a different perspective.

2. Confess that you recognize your own hostility.

3. Force yourself to stop cynical thoughts in progress.

4. Examine situations reasonably.

5. Put yourself in the other person's shoes.

6. Learn to laugh at yourself.

7. Learn to relax. Techniques such as yoga and meditation can be very useful.

8. Practice trust. Make a special effort to place trust in someone, even if in an unimportant matter.

9. Learn to listen.

10. Learn to be assertive. When difficult situations arise, assert your point of view calmly rather than reacting aggressively.

11. Pretend today is your last. Williams reflects that after people experience major illnesses, their hostility is often reduced.

12. Practice forgiving others.

The Power of Beliefs

Perhaps nothing illustrates the influence of mind over bodily function more aptly than the placebo effect. Placebo means literally "to please." A placebo is a substance that lacks intrinsic or remedial value, done or given to pacify or satisfy someone. It works because the recipient believes it has value. The placebo effect has long been considered a nuisance in medical research. It "gets in the way" of our attempts to study drugs and medical procedures. Only recently have scientists begun to investigate the implications of the placebo response as it relates to how and why we become ill. In reality, we should understand the mystery behind the placebo effect and harness its power to our advantage, much like the shamans of old.

Two cases illustrate nicely the power of the mind working through the placebo effect. Surgeons in Denmark performed an endolymphatic sac shunt on 15 patients with Meniere's disease, a disease of the inner ear with symptoms of dizziness, deafness and buzzing in the ear. These doctors also performed a placebo (sometimes called "sham") operation on 15 more patients suffering from Meniere's disease. After three years, roughly 70 percent of the subjects in each group experienced almost complete relief of their symptoms. According to the surgeons, the placebo effect was the most likely cause for improvement in these patients. The patients believed they were undergoing a beneficial surgery, thus there was a favorable outcome.[33,34]

In another instance, a patient suffering from nausea was told he would be given a new drug that would take care of his symptoms. Without his knowledge, he was given syrup of ipecac, a substance commonly used to *induce* nausea and vomiting. Within 15 minutes his symptoms disappeared.[35] Beliefs can drive the immune system so severely that some people with asthma suffer full-blown attacks as a result of looking at artificial flowers.[36]

Beliefs are critical to the placebo effect. They are critical to the healing response. When we realize that we have control over our belief systems, we can begin to exert greater control over our lives and over our health.

Giving Mirth:
Laughter May Be the Best Medicine

A short article about the health benefits of laughter appeared in a 1990 issue of *Mothering* magazine with the title *Giving Mirth*.[37] It is a curious title because it associates laughter with the birth process. *Giving birth* is a jubilant event that brings new life into the world. When we *give mirth,** we breathe new life into our cells, our mind, our outlook. Giving mirth stimulates the senses. It relieves pain, reduces stress. It helps us, if only temporarily, forget our troubles.

For some, giving mirth has literally meant bringing a new life into the world. Norman Cousins, author of *Anatomy of an Illness,* attributes his recovery from a "terminal" disease in part to laughter. Hour after hour, day after day, Cousins viewed old comedy movies. Through his laughter, he was able to give birth to a new body and mind, from what was once a diseased and dying human being.[38]

Researchers from all walks of medicine are beginning to recognize the healing powers of humor and laughter. Lee S. Berk, DHSc., M.P.H., of Loma Linda University, has discovered some of the reasons why laughter so efficiently reverses the adverse effects of stress. He has found that levels of adrenaline (epinephrine) and cortisol drop significantly following a good laugh. This results in relaxation of muscles and blood vessels and improvement in immune function. The research of Lee and others shows that humor contributes to greater optimism, cooperation and socialization—all aspects of a healthy self and a healthy society.[40]

Dr. Kathleen Dillon of Western New England College measured the levels of salivary IgA (an immunoglobulin) concentrations in students before and after viewing humorous and non-humorous video tapes. Salivary IgA is a substance that protects against viral infections. Her work showed that those viewing humorous videos increased their IgA levels, while those viewing

---

*The definition of mirth even sounds uplifting: Gladness and gaiety, especially when expressed by laughter; rejoicing or enjoyment, especially when expressed in merrymaking.[39]

non-humorous videos experienced no change. Dr. Dillon also observed that those who used humor as a means of coping with difficult life situations had higher levels of IgA initially.[41]

So, can laughter be transferred to the cells of our immune system? Are there sad and happy cells? Consider the remarks of noted author and physician Deepak Chopra: "Outfitted with a vocabulary to mirror the nervous system's in its complexity, the immune system apparently sends and receives messages that are just as diverse. In fact, if being happy, sad, thoughtful, excited, and so on all require the production of neuropeptides and neurotransmitters in our brain cells, then the immune cells must also be happy, sad, thoughtful, excited—indeed, they must be able to express the full range of 'words' that neurons do."[42]

Perhaps humor and laughter should be ranked with eating and sleeping in the realm of healthy habits.

Illness As Metaphor

Jacob was a 7-year-old boy who developed recurrent sore throats. His tonsils became swollen followed by general achiness and low-grade fever. Throat cultures were always negative and his blood counts were within normal limits. Jacob did not respond to the antibiotics prescribed by his doctors. After two weeks his sore throat would improve, only to return in another two weeks. This cycle of recurrent sore throats went on for several months. Dr. Schmidt saw Jacob and asked him to talk about his family, his school or anything else that might be on his mind. After some time spent building trust, Jacob revealed that he had recently changed schools and was having a difficult time making friends. He was also "picked on" and called names. Any effort to convey this to his parents was met with a blunt "Oh, it will get better Jacob, just try harder." He was never able to fully express the pain he experienced, nor was his distress acknowledged by his loving but overworked parents.

Dr. Schmidt counseled Jacob's parents on the importance of allowing him to speak freely of the pain and frustration he experienced at school. The parents made a special effort to encourage Jacob to talk about his experiences and helped him come up with ways to cope with his dilemma. Jacob's recurrent sore throats cleared up shortly after he was able to speak freely of his feelings.

Another patient, David, was a 35-year-old doctor. He was in the midst of a career crisis, uncertain of what he wanted to do. Medicine was unrewarding and he needed a change. His main complaint was sprained ankles. It seemed whatever he did resulted in a sprained ankle. He sprained them easily playing basketball or golf. He sprained them walking down the street, or stepping off a curb. He once stepped on a small stone and turned his ankle. The injuries were never serious, merely constant. One day while talking with a friend about his career, David realized that he had been afraid to take any steps to improve or clarify his situation. He was, in effect, paralyzed with indecision. Then it occurred to him. Perhaps his "failure to take the next step" in his career was being reflected in his body—the constantly sprained ankles. He was literally unable to take another step without spraining his ankles. Once he realized this possible connection, he took decisive measures to solve his career crisis. His ankles improved with no more episodes of injury.

What do these stories tell us? Perhaps they show that physical illness is sometimes a reflection of our inner state. Jason's story is a classic example. His sore throats would not respond until he got to the cause. Speech takes place in the throat. The pain of his psyche translated into pain in the one area that would allow him to express his hurt—the throat. We see cases like this fairly often. One only has to look.

Don't Blame the Victim

Throughout this book we have discussed hundreds of factors that seem to influence immunity and susceptibility to infection. With this comes an *apparent* onus of personal responsibility. "If I got sick, I must have done something wrong," or "I didn't do enough," or "I did too much." While personal responsibility is an important part of remaining well and preventing disease, we sometimes place too much emphasis on personal responsibility for our health based upon disease risk factors. We must recognize that some things are beyond our control, that events happen which are unknown to us, that illness occurs despite our best efforts, despite the most restrictive diets, despite the most healthful lifestyle, despite the best of intentions. We must be more understanding with ourselves and recognize that imposing guilt is not a useful motivator. We can use the information in this book as a reference point. From there we should adopt the principles espoused by Sobel and Ornstein in their book *Healthy Pleasures*. In essence, live a life of balance and find pleasure in all you do. Show compassion, love and caring for yourself. Realize that this life is a journey, and that illness is often a teacher.

Is There an Immune-Competent Personality?

Ever since the "discovery" (rediscovery, actually) that the mind affects immune function, doctors have tried to find a formula that describes the psychological profile of the immune-healthy person. Indeed, in this chapter we have explored a multitude of factors that influence our immune system. What seems to be emerging is the belief that there are no simple formulas. Rather, there is a complex interaction between attitude, behavior, traits, tendencies and events that influences immunity.

George F. Solomon, M.D., is one of the pioneers in the study of mind and immunity, known as psychoneuroimmunology. When pressed to describe the immune-competent personality, he was quick to acknowledge that there are no simple equations. He then went on to describe seven important features outlined below:[43]

1. Being in touch with your psychological and bodily needs.

2. Being able to meet those needs by assertive action.

3. Possessing coping skills, including a sense of control, that enable you to ward off depression.

4. Expressing emotions including sadness and anger.

5. Being willing to ask for and accept support from loved ones.

6. Having a sense of meaning and purpose in your work, daily activities and relationships.

7. Having a capacity for pleasure and play.

A Summary of Things to Do

1. Practice regular relaxation exercises or meditation.

2. Work at becoming more of an optimist. Optimists have healthier immune systems, suffer from fewer infections and are not as adversely affected by stressful life events. They in fact experience fewer negative events. Pessimism is reversible. Learn how to be an optimist. See *Learned Optimism* by Martin Seligman, Ph.D.

3. Guard against cynicism and hostility. If you find yourself reacting to events with hostility, stop yourself, take some deep breaths and feel how your body is responding. Death rates in people who are hostile, cynical or suspicious are four to seven times higher than in people who are not.[44,45]

4. Learn to express your feelings and emotions. Suppressed anger, sadness, grief or other emotions can lead to suppressed immunity. We all experience anger and sadness and need to express it in healthy ways. Suppressed anger has been associated with more frequent illness.

5. Take control. If you are in a situation that seems outside your control, find little things over which you can exert control. A sense of control seems to help our immune systems function more efficiently.

6. Be willing to ask for and accept support from friends and loved ones.

7. Find a sense of meaning and purpose in your relationships, work and daily activities.

8. Learn to say "no" (when you need to) when others ask for your help or services. While service and giving are important parts of a healthy life, being unable to assert yourself and claim your needs is not.

9. Keep a daily journal of your *feelings,* especially during important life events. It gives the immune system a boost that can be verified as long as six weeks after the journal-keeping has been discontinued.

10. Take classes in relaxation. Self-relaxation techniques have been shown to boost immunity, relieve pain and improve life in general.

11. Take life less seriously. As Dr. Wayne Dyer says, "Act as though what we do really matters, but realize that it does not."

12. If you are depressed, seek help from a professional. Seek out people you trust. Get moderate exercise. People suffering from depression have weakened immune systems and are more susceptible to infection.

13. Laugh as much as you can. Attend funny movies, read funny stories, socialize with funny people and try to see the humorous things in life.

14. Become more idealistic. Realists often have a more accurate view of the world, but are also more apt to be depressed, which may lead to sluggish immunity.

15. When stressful life events strike, take extra time, do relaxation exercises, write in a journal, discuss your feelings with someone you trust, stay away from junk food, take extra vitamins. During high stress periods, we are vulnerable. The extra effort spent caring for yourself will pay off.

16. Begin to view yourself as healthy. Rate your health high. Those who do actually live longer and feel better. This does not mean conscious denial or avoidance of problems that actually exist.

17. Take control of your health. Do not rely on doctors. When you use doctors, try to form a health partnership. Find a doctor whose philosophy of care is similar to your own. You will be more likely to trust his/her advice and follow through with recommendations. In such a relationship, doctors are less likely to respond negatively to your questions.

III

Natural Medicine

8

Vitamin C: Powerful Preventive and Treatment

"Vitamin C has value in preventing and treating not only the common cold and influenza, but also other viral diseases and various bacterial infections. Its main mechanism of action is through strengthening the immune system."

Linus Pauling, Ph.D.
Nobel Laureate[1]

Most of us have heard of vitamin C, or ascorbic acid. Most of us have probably tried it to see if it would help fight a cold or the flu. If it didn't work, perhaps we scorned it. Many have been helped through an infection when they took extra vitamin C. Why doesn't it work for everyone? Is it the dose taken? Is there some other catalyst that must be taken to make it work?

Enough research using double-blind, cross-over, placebo-controlled studies has been done to indicate that ascorbic acid has many valuable functions. Enhancing the immune system is the important one we want to discuss in this chapter.

Almost all of us have heard about the British sailors who got scurvy on their long sea voyages in the 16th and 17th centuries. We know that we need some fresh fruit every day or two, or we might come down with bleeding gums, depression, fatigue or a nasty infection. If we grow up and stay alive without those problems, does it mean we are getting enough vitamin C? How can we tell?

Primates such as monkeys, apes and humans cannot manufacture vitamin C from a simple sugar as can almost all other vertebrates (except guinea pigs). Apparently when we evolved as humans, our livers were so busy processing other things, and the ancient diets had so much raw fruit and vegetables anyway, evolutionary forces figured the unneeded enzyme, 1-gulonolactone oxidase, that converts glucose to ascorbic acid, could be dropped. Dr. Linus Pauling calculated that our ancient relatives, the hunters and gatherers, consumed about 600 mg of vitamin C daily in their diet of lean meat, vegetables and fruit. This amount is about 100 times the amount needed to prevent scurvy and about 10 times the current RDA (recommended daily allowance).[2]

In latitudes generally devoid of fruit, the natives discovered that to stay healthy they had to eat raw adrenal glands. They would rip open the flanks of newly felled animals, locate the kidneys and the adjacent adrenals, pull the latter out and divide them among members of the tribe. They knew if they did not eat some of this every few days, they might sicken and die. There is more vitamin C concentrated in the adrenals than in any other organ of the body. (This may hint why vitamin C is so necessary in helping prevent stress-related illness.)[3]

Different Needs

Many of us know the RDA set by the National Academy of Sciences and the National Research Council hovers around 50 to 60 mg of vitamin C daily. The scientists who arrived at this dose knew that an amount below roughly 20 mg a day could lead to scurvy. By tripling this "minimum" they reasoned that no one could get scurvy and no one would overdose. It was considered a "safe," generous and scientifically determined daily amount.

What the scientists did not realize was that there is an enormous difference between the clinical disease called scurvy and a condition of optimum health: freedom from disease, sense of well-being, ability to handle the stressors of life, the energy to awaken refreshed after seven to eight hours of quality sleep, and a cheerful, optimistic ambiance. The researchers believed that if you did not have scurvy, you did not need any extra vitamin C. They were convinced that any improvement in health or mental attitude attributed to the intake of vitamin C must be due to other factors.

Dr. Joseph Beasley in *The Kellogg Report* cited the work of the late biochemist Dr. Roger Williams, who in 1950 pointed out how different we all are. Individual requirements for a nutrient may not be met by diet. Chronic disease results from these unmet requirements.[4] Dr. Frederick Klenner suggested the following reasons why we all have different needs for vitamin C:

- age
- alcohol
- exposure to pesticides
- tobacco
- trauma
- emotional stress
- kidney threshold
- absorption
- acidity or alkalinity
- physiological stress
- poor vitamin storage
- habits
- drugs
- carbon monoxide
- sleep
- infection
- surgery
- loss in stools
- differences in body chemistry
- climate
- weight

The National Academy of Sciences gave little consideration to these differences when determining the RDA. However, their assertion that 60 mg of vitamin C is enough for all of us has been challenged by recent findings. Smokers were found to need 200 mg of vitamin C daily just to maintain the same blood level of non-smokers getting only 60 mg of vitamin C a day.[5] This suggests that exposure to chemicals or differences in lifestyle alter our vitamin C needs.

More striking are findings of a recent symposium sponsored by the National Cancer Institute. In an evaluation of 47 studies of vitamin C and cancer, 380 mg of vitamin C daily was found to be protective against cancer of the lung, larynx, oral cavity, esophagus, stomach, colon, rectum, pancreas, bladder, cervix, endometrium and breast, as well as childhood brain tumor. People in the top 25 percent of vitamin C intake have approximately one-half the cancer risk of those in the bottom 25 percent of vitamin C intake.[6]

This work and more suggests that our individual needs for vitamin C (and other nutrients) varies widely, and that increasing our intake of vitamin C is protective against some of humankind's most devastating ills.

On the Wrong Course

During the 1930s, after vitamin C was synthesized in the laboratory, many clinicians began to accumulate anecdotal evidence that substantial doses of vitamin—many times the RDA—were able to make people feel well or get well. It was also during the 1930s that chemists were beginning to extract and synthesize drugs that could be shown to have antibiotic properties against infections, especially bacterial infections.

The Germans first synthesized Prontosol, a type of sulfa drug. The race was on. Penicillin was manufactured in the early 1940s from a common mold. Mycins were discovered that could be extracted from plants and molds. The benefits of vitamin C as a safe therapeutic agent did not capture the attention of the world as did the miracles that the manufactured drugs provided. The promise of modern medicine was becoming a reality. One of the most potent healing substances known, vitamin C, was relegated to archives of medical journals and the clinics of a few noble physicians.

Dr. Beasley points out that the drug era shifted funding to the development of new drugs despite the promise of nutrition.[7] In the last few years, the National Cancer Institute has spent only about 1 percent of its funds on nutritional research: this despite the statement of the deputy director in 1977 before the Senate Select Committee that about 60 percent of cancers in women and 40 percent of cancers in men appear to be related to diet. The role of vitamin C in the treatment of infections was almost forgotten.

Vitamin C and Infectious Disease

Frederick Klenner, M.D., was impressed back in the 1930s with the curative effects of vitamin C. He experimented on his own children and patients and found he could stop diseases—especially the viral contagious diseases of children—within minutes or hours with large doses of vitamin C. He was one of the first to detect decreased levels of vitamin C in the blood of patients with infectious diseases; the longer the disease lasted and the more severe the symptoms, the lower the level of vitamin C. It seemed obvious to him that many such diseases were due to a sub-scurvy condition in the victim. He felt that patients with these low levels of vitamin C were at risk for viral encephalitis and possible coma and death. He knew that vitamin C was needed to make the intercellular substance that holds the capillaries together. Those spaces could be weakened, and the virus or bacteria could slip through to the brain. Capillaries become fragile when the level of vitamin C in the blood drops to one mg per liter. This was known and published in the 1940s.[8,9,10,11]

In the 1960s, Dr. Archie Kalokerinos, a physician with the Australian Health Service, noticed that when Australian Aborigine children were given DPT immunization shots, every other child died. Kalokerinos believed that these children had truncated immune systems because of their impoverished diet: no fresh food, but plenty of white bread and canned goods. So, very logically, he provided vitamin C to them in the dose of 100 mg/day/month of age. For example, a six-month-old would get 600 mg daily. A one-year-old would receive 1,200 mg/day and a two-year-old 2,400 mg/day. The result at the next immunization go-around? Nobody died.[12] Others have since repeated this work. Some doctors now give 1,000 mg of vitamin C to a child at the time of vaccination. (For parents unable to talk their doctor into this method, they can give the infant or child 1,000 mg of C, 1,000 mg of calcium and 100 mg of B_6 by mouth on the day before, the day of and the day after the shot. All very safe and quite effective.)

Another report, this one published in 1950, showed vitamin C was helpful in caring for childhood diseases. According to an article in the *Journal of the American Medical Association,* 90 children with whooping cough (pertussis) were treated using intravenous vitamin C, oral vitamin C or vaccine. Vitamin C dosage began at 500 mg daily and was reduced by 100 mg each day until a daily dose of 100 mg was reached. Thereafter, children were maintained on 100 mg per day until they recovered. Children receiving intravenous vitamin C were well in 15 days. Those treated with oral vitamin C were well in 25 days. while those treated with vaccine were well in an average of 34 days. What was perhaps most impressive was that in roughly 75 percent of cases in which vitamin C was started in the catarrhal stage, "the spasmodic stage was wholly prevented."[13]

Much research has been done on the use of vitamin C and viral infections. There have also been reports of vitamin C and bacterial infections. In one study a concentration of one milligram per deciliter prevented the growth in culture of the tuberculosis bacterium. Vitamin C has also been shown to inactivate other bacteria including those causing typhoid fever, staphylococcal infections and tetanus. It has also been shown to inactivate the *toxins* of tetanus, dysentery, diphtheria and staphylococcus.[14,15,16]

Vitamin C probably works by having a direct effect on certain viruses and bacteria and also by boosting certain aspects of the immune system. Dr. Pauling has reported that vitamin C is needed for effective phagocytosis by white blood cells.[17] Phagocytosis is the process by which white cells (leukocytes) gobble up bacteria. When white cells are high in vitamin C, they gobble heartily. When they are low, they don't. Members of a Scottish population in good health on an ordinary Scottish diet were found to have slightly more vitamin C in their leukocytes than was needed for proper phagocytic activity. However, after contracting colds, the level of vitamin C fell to half the original level and remained low for several days. (This renders one more susceptible to secondary bacterial infection.) Each was given 250 mg of vitamin C daily, but this was not enough to raise the leukocyte levels of vitamin C sufficiently to permit phagocytosis. It was discovered that *six grams* per day was required at the beginning of the cold and one gram per day thereafter to maintain phagocytosis at the appropriate level.[18] Antibiotics are often given to people with viral infections in an effort to prevent secondary bacterial infection. According to Drs. Cathcart, Pauling and Cameron, vitamin C can be helpful in limiting the development of secondary bacterial infection—probably by stimulating phagocytosis.

In 1977, Dr. J. Asfora carried out one of the best studies on the therapeutic benefit of vitamin C. One hundred thirty-three medical students, physicians or clinic patients were given either

1,000 mg vitamin C (two tablets, three times daily) or a placebo. Some began taking the tablets on the first day of the cold, others on the second day and others on the third day. Those taking vitamin C fared much better with regard to cold symptoms. Most interesting was the finding that those who took vitamin C on the first day of the cold suffered fewer bacterial complications than those not taking vitamin C or those starting vitamin C on the second or third day of symptoms. Only 13 percent of those who began vitamin C on the first day developed secondary bacterial infection. This was in comparison to 20 percent who began the vitamin on the second day, 41 percent who began on the third day and 39 percent who took the placebo.[19]

Vitamin C also has a direct effect on antibodies—the proteins formed by white cells (B-cells) that enable the bodily defenses to recognize and destroy bacteria. After giving healthy college students one gram of vitamin C per day for 75 days, a significant rise occurred in the kind of antibodies needed to fight bacteria and viruses.[20]

With the emergence of an ever-increasing array of infectious diseases from hepatitis B and C, to AIDS and pneumocystis, the value of vitamin C grows. Dr. Smith once attended a sick, semi-comatose young man with the AIDS complication of pneumonia. His skin was blue-tinged despite six to eight liters of oxygen per minute flowing into him by nasal catheter. Dr. Smith administered five grams of vitamin C into each of four muscles (deltoids and glutei). The patient was so obtunded he did not know that the shots had been given without local anesthetic (intramuscular vitamin C is painful without procaine). He was better in eight hours—still sick of course, but he needed only four liters of oxygen and was home in a week.

There is a famous story of a little three-year-old girl who developed encephalitis after a flu-like disease. She had lain in the hospital for a week like a vegetable, receiving her meals a sip at a time. Her father asked the doctor about vitamin C.

"Nonsense. If you give her those vitamins, you can find another doctor for her," was the stern reply.

"Would it be alright if I gave her some ice cream instead of the hospital gelatin?" the father asked obsequiously. That was fine.

The father came back daily with her favorite flavor, vanilla, but with a teaspoon of vitamin C powder (4,000 mg) in each dishful. In just four days the child was sitting up, eating and moving about. She was discharged in another few days. The doctor signed out the chart as a "spontaneous recovery from encephalitis."

Vitamin C in Action: What It Can Do

Research has demonstrated that ascorbic acid acts as an oxidizing agent, a reducing agent, an anticlotting agent, an antihistamine (stabilizes mast cells containing histamine) and, of course, as an anti-infectious agent. For the immune system, it supports stressed-out adrenal glands, stimulates the production of interferon, and enhances the antiviral and antibacterial action of white blood cells. A deficiency of vitamin C will produce a decrease in the T-cells needed by the immune system.

Vitamin C has other related benefits. It is the most powerful protector against free radicals known. Free radicals are highly reactive chemical species that can destroy proteins, fats, DNA and cell membranes, contribute to aging and cause cancer. Free radicals are present throughout the environment and also are produced within the body. No substance protects the body from damage like vitamin C. Vitamin C protects against toxic metals like mercury, lead, cadmium, excess chromium and aluminum. It protects against excess x-radiation and ultraviolet radiation. When mice with large malignant skin tumors were exposed to ultraviolet radiation, those with the highest levels of vitamin C in their diet were least affected by the radiation—the incidence of tumors in the high vitamin C animals went down.[21]

Vitamin C is essential for collagen formation; this is the substance that holds all our body tissues together. Vitamin C counteracts the damage of cigarette smoke. Cigarette smoking uses about 100 mg of vitamin C per cigarette. Vitamin C helps those taking oral contraceptives, cortisone and some antibiotics. Use of aspirin and alcohol will reduce the storage of vitamin C in the body.

Vitamin C proceeds into each cell and interferes with the production of new viruses. The cells rupture and die, so there are no virus particles to infect new cells. From the research done in the

1930s Dr. Klenner concluded, "The degree of neutralization in a virus infection will be in proportion to the concentration of the vitamin and the length of time it is employed."[22] This is the best explanation for those who have been disappointed in their response to vitamin C therapy: not enough C for too short a period. The vitamin C combines with the virus, bacteria or chemical substance and a new compound is formed, which must be oxidized by more C. Hence, vitamin C therapy must be continuous and prolonged beyond the initial response.

Dr. Emanuel Cheraskin was able to show that the higher the daily dose of vitamin C, the fewer symptoms one reported. He also showed that vitamin C was able to improve the functional capacity of white blood cells. (Dr. Klenner said that a white blood cell without C is like a soldier without bullets.)[23] When one gets sick, for whatever reason, the sickness itself acts as a stressor to further deplete the immune system. Dr. Klenner was able to see the progress of a simple but prolonged cold lead to a complication such as otitis, bronchitis or encephalitis. His motivating slogan: "Give vitamin C while pondering the diagnosis."

Two to five grams of vitamin C daily will increase the activity of lymphocytes and improve the migration and mobility of leukocytes. During a serious infection, vitamin C is mobilized to fight the intruders. This depletion can make one more vulnerable to allergies, arthritis, depression and other maladies. No matter what the infection, one should take vitamin C during and after.

The Right Dose

Dr. Robert Cathcart recently championed the benefits of large doses of vitamin C. After some clinical experience, he was able to categorize the sickness into the need for vitamin C: "This patient has a 20,000 mg (20 g) cold" or "She needs 100 grams for her mono." The more ill patients seemed, the more vitamin C they required and the more often the dose needed repeating. He learned from Klenner who said, "If a patient does not respond to vitamin C, it means he was not given enough."[24]

In one study, one gram of vitamin C daily reduced the duration and severity of colds by 37 percent. Higher doses are usually recommended and produce a more pronounced improvement. In a study using matched pairs of twins, those receiving vitamin C got 19 percent fewer colds, the duration was 38 percent shorter, severity was 22 percent less and the intensity was 20 percent less. An intravenous infusion of seven grams of vitamin C nearly eliminated hepatitis due to transfusion passage of the virus.

Much important research has been done on finding the optimum dose of vitamin C by Emanuel Cheraskin, M.D., D.M.D.. He correlated symptoms and complaints in students, dentists and their spouses with the daily doses of vitamin C they were swallowing. He also pointed out that in the *Journal of the American Medical Association* in 1985, somewhere between 3 and 50 percent of the population had signs of scurvy, and 17 to 72 percent had suboptimal intake of vitamin C or sub-clinical scurvy. His multiple findings: In those who took at least 400 mg of vitamin C daily, the incidence of respiratory symptoms was fewer than in those who took less than 400 mg daily. The higher the intake of vitamin C, the fewer cardiovascular symptoms. Since fatigue is the first symptom that patients have when they are coming down with scurvy (it takes 90 days to get a full-blown case), those who were taking less than 400 mg had many complaints of fatigue, while those getting at least 400 mg of vitamin C had almost no fatigue. Eighty-one subjects who got less than 100 mg of vitamin C had a fatigability score twice that of those who ingested more than 400 mg of vitamin C daily. In addition, there were more skin symptoms in those on less than 400 mg daily.[25]

Healthy people can take up to 10 grams daily with no side effects. If they ingest more, they are likely to develop watery bowel movements. There is no set amount that is considered just right, as there is a 400 percent difference in the amount of vitamin C absorbed by human subjects. Most patients and doctors individualize the dose depending on bowel tolerance. When the daily dose is found that begins to loosen the stools, that is the saturation dose. The next day the dose is reduced about 10 percent to the dose that does not cause this rectal irritation.

To find the right dose for you will take some experimentation. Linus Pauling takes 18,000 mg daily. If you're healthy, you probably require much less on a daily basis, but during times of illness, you may require more than Dr. Pauling. The key is to identify the amount that is optimum for you, recognizing that the need can change with seasons, sleep, illness, stress, eating habits and numerous factors mentioned earlier.

Vitamin C and Animals

One reason Nobel Laureate Linus Pauling became interested in studying vitamin C was the extraordinary finding that most animals manufacture 10,000 mg per day, when one corrects for human body weight. In testing animals that can manufacture their own vitamin C when stressed or sick, Klenner found that animals do not stop at the ridiculously low level established by the government agencies. The animals, when stressed, manufacture the equivalent of a human swallowing 15 grams of C each day that the stressors are operative. Dr. Klenner pointed out that "the physiological requirements in man are no different from other mammals capable of carrying out their synthesis of vitamin C."

Research in 1934 found that the vitamin C level in the adrenal glands was greatly reduced in animals succumbing to polio, showing that even animals that manufacture their own vitamin C can be at risk.[26] Canine pups suffering from distemper, an often fatal disease, can almost be assured of survival if given adequate vitamin C.

Deficiency Signs

Deficiency of vitamin C probably affects almost all body systems. The most obvious and well-researched symptoms are listed below. Not all symptoms need be present.

Bleeding gums	Easy bruising
Fatigue	Tiredness
Malaise	Loose teeth
Depression	Frequent infections
Irritability	Poor wound healing

Is Vitamin C Safe?

Vitamin C is believed to be one of the safest substances that humans ingest. However, many in the medical community continue to criticize the use of vitamin C based on what now appear to be erroneous conclusions. Critics of the use of vitamin C generally cite a litany of complaints that focuses on four areas:

- Vitamin C is said to increase destruction of vitamin B_{12} contributing to the loss of this vitamin.
- Vitamin C is said to contribute to iron overload.
- A condition dubbed "rebound scurvy" is said to occur when consumption of high doses of vitamin C is abruptly stopped.
- Vitamin C is said to contribute to the formation of kidney stones.

It is beyond the scope of this book to discuss each of these topics in great depth. However, a brief response to each of these assertions is warranted. We should first note that there has never been a report in the medical literature of poisoning, death or hospitalization related to vitamin C use. This stands in stark contrast to the many poisonings and hospitalizations related to over-the-counter and prescription drugs reported each year.

In 1987, Dr. Jerry M. Rivers, then of Cornell University, wrote a paper published in the *Annals of the New York Academy of Sciences* entitled "Safety of High-Level Vitamin C Ingestion." In this extensive review of the available research, he comments on each of the assertions mentioned above.[27]

Regarding B_{12} destruction: "The evidence has consistently demonstrated that vitamin B_{12} in food and the body is not destroyed by ascorbic acid."

Regarding iron overload: ". . . it appears highly unlikely that large doses of the vitamin would lead to excessive iron accumulation in the body."

Regarding rebound scurvy: "The claim that abrupt cessation of large doses of ascorbic acid will lead to scurvy because of conditioning [rebound scurvy] is not supported by the evidence."

Regarding formation of kidney stones: "It seems safe to conclude that ingestion of large quantities of the vitamin [C] does not constitute a risk factor for calcium oxalate stone formation in most healthy persons." He goes on to state that ". . . recurrent stone formers should avoid high-dose ascorbate intake. Patients with renal impairment and patients on chronic hemodialysis should also be advised not to ingest large quantities of the vitamin."

Dr. D. Hornig of the Department of Human Nutrition and Health, Hoffmann-La Roche & Co. Ltd., further remarks on the safety concerns of vitamin C. He states, "There is not a single case reported in the literature demonstrating clinically that ascorbic acid causes kidney stones." As for rebound scurvy, Hornig reports on a study his group conducted in collaboration with the prestigious Karolinska Hospital in Stockholm, Sweden, in which 5 grams of vitamin C was given daily, then stopped. According to Hornig, "The results indicate no such effect [i.e., no rebound scurvy] on the basis of plasma, leukocyte, or urine ascorbic acid concentrations."[28]

Nutrition researchers Emanual Cheraskin, M.D., and W. Marshall Rinsdorf, D.M.D., in their book *The Vitamin C Connection* state rather bluntly, "As for the other grim tales—ranging from B[12] deficiency to kidney stones—let us simply say that the reports of C's evils are *greatly* exaggerated! Indeed, in the absence of scientific evidence more convincing than the negative studies we're aware of and have mentioned in this chapter, we are inclined to think C is innocent of the bad effects ascribed to it."[29]

Another final complaint levied at vitamin C is the vitamin's ability to alter certain blood tests. The solution is quite simple. If you're having blood work done, notify your doctor that you have been taking vitamin C. If you know in advance that you will be having a blood test done, simply stop taking vitamin C for several days before the test.

The Vindication of Vitamin C

Nobel Prize winner Linus Pauling, Ph.D., has received decades of undeserved criticism over his views about vitamin C. His early work surrounding vitamin C as an anticancer agent was perhaps met with the greatest scorn of all. Despite all the published research he presented to make his case, allopathic doctors refused to budge from their comfortable antivitamin stance. Recently, the tables have begun to turn. In 1991, the prestigious National Cancer Institute (NCI) convened a conference on vitamin C and cancer.

According to Dr. Gladys Block, an epidemiologist in the Division of Cancer Prevention and control at NCI, vitamin C has been shown to be protective against cancer of the lung, larynx, oral cavity, esophagus, stomach, colon, rectum, pancreas, bladder, cervix, endometrium and breast, as well as childhood brain tumor. Of a total of 47 studies, 34 found vitamin C to be protective against these cancers. According to researchers, "If chance alone was at work here, out of these 47 studies undertaken only one or two would have proven to be statistically significant." More dramatic, people in the top 25 percent of vitamin C intake have roughly one-half the cancer risk of those in the lowest 25 percent of vitamin C intake.[30]

Morton A. Klein, health economist and former consultant to the Department of Health, Education and Welfare, spoke with many of the doctors and scientists after the conference. Many of them were so intrigued with the findings presented at the conference that "they intended to increase their personal daily intake of vitamin C to 1,000 mg/day or more."[31]

Now that such impressive work has been released on the benefits of this simple but remarkable vitamin, perhaps the pioneering work of Drs. Klenner, Cathcart and others regarding the use of vitamin C and infections will be given a fresh and objective look. When this occurs it is likely that vitamin C will be found to be one of the most efficient antibacterial, antiviral and immune-boosting substances available.

Basic Rules for Vitamin C Use

Vitamin C is vital to a variety of body functions. Most humans probably don't get enough of this vitamin. Certainly during times of increased vitamin C need, most humans never have their needs met. How do we meet our daily need and know when there is increased need?

Vitamin C: Powerful Preventive and Treatment

Remember, vitamin C has a very wide margin of safety. It is not going to harm anyone to take 500 mg every day. This would be considered a bare minimum. Dr. Pauling recommends between 1,000 and 18,000 mg daily, while Dr. Roger Williams suggested about 2,500 mg daily. During times of infection this can easily be increased to 10,000 or 20,000 mg daily. A physician administering intravenous ascorbic acid for infectious mononucleosis might use 100 grams (1g = 1,000 mg) or more daily until symptoms improve. There has been virtually no toxicity associated with these higher doses, especially when used over the short term.

Intravenous is the most effective means of administering ascorbic acid (in combination with calcium and magnesium salts), but it is not always necessary or practical. When vitamin C is taken by mouth, it is best to take frequent doses over time rather than fewer large doses. A substantial amount of vitamin C can be absorbed through the mouth, so vitamin C lozenges are a good way to obtain the vitamin. (But brush your teeth afterward. The acid could dissolve your tooth enamel.) Powdered vitamin C is more efficiently utilized than tablets. As a daily supplement, tablets are fine. During illness, powder may be best.

Dr. Robert Cathcart has championed the concept of bowel tolerance to determine the correct dose of vitamin C. Take large doses until the stools become loose. Then reduce the dosage gradually until diarrhea ceases. This will be the optimum dose. For example, if the flu has been going around and you feel symptoms coming on, begin to take vitamin C in doses of roughly 20 grams per day. If you experience softening of the stool, reduce the dose to 18 grams. If the stool is still loose, reduce the dose to 15 grams and so on. Once the stool is firm, you will have reached the right dose for you at that time. When you are over the flu, 15 grams may produce diarrhea because your need has decreased.

A small percentage of people say they are allergic to vitamin C. In most cases, it is probably an allergy to one of the excipients used in manufacture of the tablet. It may also indicate a sensitivity to corn, since some brands of vitamin C are derived from corn. If you react adversely, try another brand of vitamin C. If you still react, get some vitamin C that is not derived from corn.

If you use vitamin C to manage an illness and don't feel yourself improving to your satisfaction, you probably have not taken enough vitamin C. It may also be that you need other nutrients or that you have a concurrent condition that requires medical attention. Antibiotics can be useful for some types of infections, but even when antibiotics are used, vitamin C should be supplemented to boost immunity and assist in combating the invaders.

Vitamin C is among the most powerful antioxidants. However, the body uses a number of other antioxidant nutrients that work in concert with vitamin C. Whenever you take vitamin C it is important that you also take vitamin E, beta-carotene and other antioxidants.

Vitamin C is never taken "in vain." It is a substance used actively by the body. If you are using vitamin C and do not notice dramatic improvement, do not discontinue. By nature, vitamin C levels fall during infection. At the very least, you will be keeping up with that which is being lost.

The advice offered to physicians by Dr. Klenner can also be offered to non-physicians: "Give vitamin C while pondering the diagnosis." If you feel an illness coming on and you are unsure whether it is viral, bacterial, allergy, dry air or trauma, take vitamin C. It will always do some good.

9

Boosting Immunity Naturally: Complementary Treatments Old and New

"It is the body that is the hero, not science, not antibiotics, not machines or new devices."

Ronald J. Glasser, M.D.
The Body is the Hero[1]

By now we hope to have made it clear that a major pitfall of the "antibiotics only" approach to infection is that it gives little regard to the immunity of the host, natural elimination mechanisms and healing of tissues. A beautiful feature of holistic medical approaches such as herbology, homeopathy or use of essential oils (often referred to as aromatherapy) is that not only do the substances used often kill or inhibit organisms directly, but they also stimulate immune function, encourage elimination of bacterial toxins, stimulate kidney and liver function, and speed recovery. With these approaches, we often have the best of both worlds.

In this section we review the use of herbs, essential oils, homeopathic medicine and hands-on healing as means to enhance or balance immune function. This is not meant to be an extensive presentation, but an introduction to approaches that have been effectively used for centuries and are growing in popularity today. Though none of these methods represent a panacea, they are extremely effective when properly used.

We use the term "complementary treatments" to show that they complement, enhance and support natural body functions. They can also be used to complement or enhance other forms of medicine such as the allopathic use of antibiotics or surgery.

Herbal Medicine: Is the Cure in the Jungle?

While many Western allopathic doctors would have us believe there is no value to herbal medicine, the evidence shows otherwise. Seventy-five percent of drugs are based on knowledge of plant substances. One-fourth of all prescription drugs contain one or more plant-derived ingredients. For instance, childhood leukemia once had a mortality rate of 80 percent. Today there is an 80 percent survival rate thanks to the drug vincristine, derived from the rosy periwinkle.

According to Technology Management Group of New Haven, Connecticut, there are more than 200 companies and research firms investigating plants for new drugs.[2] This suggests there is more than a casual interest in plant substances. So why do we hear negative press about herbal medicine, and why do we hear herbs denigrated by the medical establishment? The main reason is ignorance. Most health professionals and media people who comment on herbal medicine have little or no knowledge of the subject. The second reason is that herbal medicines cannot be patented, thus there is no incentive for the medical-industrial complex to develop them. On the other hand, drugs derived from plant extracts can be synthesized, patented and sold to the tune of millions of dollars. Therefore, the FDA has provided no incentive to develop herbal medicines with their full complement of active substances. Instead, it provides incentive to develop only the active constituent "believed" to have therapeutic activity.

Below is a discussion of common herbs used to boost immunity during bacterial, viral and parasitic illness.

Citrus Seed Extract. Derived from grapefruit seeds, this supplement has been used by the food industry for the past decade because of its antimicrobial activity. It is used in food to prevent spoilage. It has also been used outside of the United States for many years in treating human illness. Only recently has it been used here for medical purposes. It is a very potent antibacterial and antifungal. It is one of the first choices in treating *Candida albicans* infection of the intestines and is used for other intestinal disorders. Because of its powerful action, the Pasteur Institute in France is testing the extract on the HIV virus associated with AIDS.

Echinacea. This is one of the most widely used and heavily studied immune-boosting herbs in the world. According to Dr. Daniel B. Mowrey in *The Scientific Validation of Herbal Medicine,* "Laboratory studies show that the herb increases the ability of white cells to surround and destroy bacterial and viral invaders in the blood. It stimulates the lymphatic system to clean up waste material and toxins, and it has definite antimicrobial activity."[3] In his book *Echinacea: Nature's Immune Enhancer,* herbalist Steven Foster summarizes many scientific studies conducted on the use of echinacea in viral and bacterial infections. This herb has been used effectively in bronchitis, whooping cough, tonsillitis, candida infections and viral upper respiratory infections. It was also shown to be a 30 percent more potent T-cell stimulator than the most potent T-cell stimulator known at this time.[4]

Garlic. Garlic has been used to treat illness for thousands of years. It is a powerful antiviral, antifungal and antibacterial herb. It has been proven effective against staph and strep, *E. coli, Salmonella, Klebsiella, Proteus, Candida albicans* and other microbes.[5] In an impressive study conducted in China, 11 patients with the usually-fatal cryptococcal meningitis were given garlic extract by mouth or by injection. Side effects were minimal and all patients recovered.[6] Garlic has been shown to be more effective than penicillin for sore throats.[7] In fact, a study appeared in the *Journal of the American Chemical Society* showing that one milligram of the major garlic constituent, allicin, is equal to 15 standard units of penicillin.[8]

Garlic is helpful in preventing colds and influenza and is useful in other forms of viral illness. While garlic is widely used and extremely helpful, there are certain conditions in which garlic may not be the best choice. In people with "hot" conditions, garlic is often not appropriate. This includes certain forms of arthritis and the treatment of people who are hot, energetic and quick-tempered. Garlic is also not the best choice in conditions of burnout or exhaustion accompanied by insomnia and lack of energy.

Goldenseal. Goldenseal has a long history of use in infections including bacterial, viral, fungal and parasitic. Staph, strep, *E. coli*, *Vibrio cholera*, *Giardia lamblia*, *Entamoeba histolytica* and even the tuberculosis bacterium have proven sensitive to this herb.[9] Since goldenseal has strong antibiotic properties, it should not be used for extended periods because it can cause disruption of the normal inhabitants of the intestines.

Goldenseal should not be used when there are digestive symptoms or, since it is a central nervous system stimulant, when there is nervousness, anxiety or excitability. This herb is considered "cooling," the opposite effect of garlic. It should be avoided in people who tend to have aversion to cold drinks, cold surroundings, who need extra covers or who have cold hands and feet. It should also be avoided during pregnancy.

Licorice Root. Licorice root is antibacterial, antiviral and anti-inflammatory. In one Japanese study, strains of *Staphylococcus aureus* that proved resistant to penicillin and streptomycin were inactivated by licorice root extract. This herb also stimulates production of interferon, a compound produced by the body to defeat viruses.[10] Inflammation often accompanies infection, and licorice has been found to be an effective anti-inflammatory agent.

Shiitake Mushrooms. *Lentinus edodes,* or shiitake mushroom, is a powerful immune stimulant. It has been shown to stimulate T-cell activity, macrophage phagocytosis and the body's production of interferon. It is able to increase resistance to bacterial, viral and parasitic fungal infection.[11] This herb is often used as a preventive in people susceptible to viral and bacterial infection. The shiitake mushroom purchased in grocery stores does not provide enough of the active constituents to be clinically effective. For medicinal purposes, the mycelia of the mushroom are gathered and concentrated.

Health professionals who use herbs commonly utilize those listed above to manage infection or treat immune deficiency. They usually use these in combination with other herbs to optimize results.

The following report illustrates the beauty, simplicity, and effectiveness of summoning the plant world during infection. The case involves Dr. Susan Esch, who practices in St. Paul, Minnesota. Dr. Esch had experienced a puncture wound of the finger while gardening. After carefully cleaning the area, she began to use several natural remedies. The remedies seemed to keep the infection from spreading to the bloodstream, but the finger was obviously not improved. She then went on a course of antibiotic, believing a strong-acting medication might solve the problem. After one course of antibiotic there was no improvement in the finger, which was now noticeably infected.

She then consulted with a colleague who had been in practice some 50 years. He suggested she use a flax seed poultice made by placing ½ cup of flax seeds in water and cooking until the mixture reached the consistency of oatmeal. This mucus-like material was put on a gauze pad and placed over the infected wound. The poultice was replaced once daily (four times daily was suggested for serious infections or tumors). After four days, Dr. Esch felt a pulling sensation at the site of the puncture, as though something was being drawn out. The next day she noticed something sticking out of the puncture site. She grasped it with a tweezers and pulled out a one and one-half inch plant stem compressed into an accordion configuration. Attached to the bottom of the stem was a tiny sac of pus. Dr. Esch cleaned the wound with hydrogen peroxide and it healed in short order.

For more information on herbal medicine see:

The Scientific Validation of Herbal Medicine by Daniel B. Mowrey (Cormorant Books, 1986).

The Way of Herbs by Michael Tierra (New York: Pocket, 1990).

The Healing Herbs by Michael Castleman (Emmaus, PA: Rodale, 1991).

Essential Plant Oils:
A Medical Breakthrough for Infection?

European physicians have been carrying out extensive research into the use of plant oils in the treatment of infections. Plant oils are biologically active components of the plant that are extracted through a process called distillation or, in the case of citrus oil, pressing. One of the advantages essential oils have over antibiotics is that bacteria do not develop resistance to essential oils. It seems almost too good to be true, but it appears that many of the antibacterial plant oils work by interfering with the bacteria's ability to breathe.[12] The bacteria literally suffocate to death.

Another advantage to essential oils is that some actually stimulate immune function. Thus, some are directly bactericidal, fungicidal and virucidal while others boost immune defenses.

The therapeutic use of essential oils is applied through a system of treatment known as aromatherapy. The term "aromatherapy" is used because these oils easily evaporate and it is often the vapors (or aroma) that have therapeutic benefit. For example, eucalyptus oil can be inhaled to reduce spasmodic coughing. The oil of *Inula graveolens* can be inhaled to treat heavy bronchial congestion. Essential oils are also easily absorbed through the skin. Oil of lavender, which has many active chemical constituents that boost immunity, can be rubbed on the body whenever a cold, flu or bacterial illness is going around. The oil is absorbed through the skin into the bloodstream and boosts immunity. (These oils are absorbed through the skin within 20 to 40 minutes—100 times faster than water.)[14] Illness can often be prevented in this way.

Drs. E. Gildemeister and F.R. Hoffmann wanted to test the antibacterial and antifungal activity of common essential plant oils. They used phenol as their reference point and assigned it an arbitrary reference value of 1.0. If a plant oil was less antibacterial or antifungal than phenol, it would receive a number less than 1. If the plant oil was more antibacterial or antifungal than phenol, it would receive a value greater than 1.0. Recall that phenol is an antiseptic substance found in Lysol®, Pinesol®, Chloraseptic® throat spray and other commonly used items. The findings were quite a surprise. All the oils tested proved to be more active antimicro-bials than phenol. Oil of lavender, very safe, pleasant and widely used, scored 1.6. Oil of oregano received a score of 21. Below is a list of the oils tested in reference to phenol.[15]

Phenol. 1.0

Lavender 1.6

Lemon 2.2

Citral. 5.0

Clove. 8.0

Thyme 13

Oregano 21

The essential oil of *Thymus vulgaris* was tested against com-mon infectious organisms such as *Candida albicans, Klebsiella pneumoniae* and *Staphylococcus aureus* and was found to be an effective antibacterial.[16] Dr. H. Rommelt and his associates showed in 1988 that essential oils in inhaled air, even in small concentra-tions, increased bronchial secretion, thinned mucus and significant-ly reduced bronchial spasms.[17] An Indian study published in 1971 showed that lemongrass oil was more effective against *Staph. aureus* than penicillin and streptomycin.[18]

According to Kurt Schnaubelt, Ph.D.,* a leading U.S. re-searcher and educator in the chemistry and therapeutic applica-tion of essential oils, infectious illness is an area where essential oils have been most effectively applied. He has reported on numer-ous studies that have shown essential oils to directly stimulate specific immunoglobulins—what we typically think of as antibod-ies designed to fight infection. Tea tree *(Melaleuca a.),* Thyme *(Thymus v.)* and other oils are able to boost immunity by enhanc-ing the body's own manufacture of gamma-globulin. According to one study published by essential oil researcher H. M. Gattefossé, all oils tested showed the ability to stimulate phagocytosis to some degree.[19]

---

* Dr. Kurt Schnaubelt, Pacific Institute of Aromatherapy, P.O. Box 6723, San Rafael, California 94903 (415) 479-9121.

As we discussed in Chapter 2, more than $500 million are spent each year on antibiotics to treat ear infections in children. In one study, doctors found a mixture of essential oils to be superior to that of the antibiotic neomycin. They treated 170 children with eardrops consisting of borneol (20 percent) and walnut oil, and another group of 108 children with drops of the antibiotic neomycin. All children in both groups suffered from purulent otitis media—infection of the middle ear with pus. The borneol-walnut oil mixture was effective in 98 percent of children while neomycin was effective in 84 percent. The researchers concluded, "Due to its simple composition, significant therapeutic effects and nontoxic reactions, the borneol-walnut oil has been proven a promising external remedy for the treatment of purulent otitis media."[20]

Treatment of bladder infections in women is an area where essential oils perhaps have their most dramatic impact. Dr. Schnaubelt describes cases of acute bladder infections in which the symptoms are reduced in minutes to hours using the oil of *Melaleuca alternifolia* (tea tree oil). Even in cases of chronic cystitis, a combination of tea tree and thyme oil is often all that is required to remedy the condition. Dr. Paul Belaiche, of the Medical Faculty at the Université de Paris Nord, "has achieved a success rate of better than 80 percent with herbal treatment of several thousand women suffering from cystitis who had failed to respond to conventional treatment."[21]

Below is a list of some common essential oils and their use in infectious illness.

Tea tree oil. The scientific name is *Melaleuca alternifolia*. This is one of the most widely used of all essential oils. It is antibacterial and antifungal. In World War II, it was blended with machine cutting oils to protect workers against infections of cuts produced by metal filings. Tea tree oil is being used by some physicians to effectively treat bladder infections in women. It is also being used to treat vaginal and intestinal candidiasis. This is one of the safest essential oils and can be used for extended periods with little irritation.

Oil of thyme, oregano and savory. These oils are often considered together because they are similar in their potent action during infection. They are bactericidal, fungicidal, virucidal and also stimulate the immune system by their effect on immunoglobulins. They are used in infections of the throat, respiratory tract, digestive tract and urogenital tract. These oils are quite potent, so only small amounts are required. They are not to be taken for more than a week unless directed by your doctor. (Author and aromatherapy researcher Robert Tisserand does not consider regular thyme oil safe for home use.)[22]

Thyme (thuyanol). Different from the thyme mentioned above, this chemotype of *Thymus vulgaris* has been shown to inhibit many microorganisms including *Klebsiella pneumoniae, E. coli* and *Candida albicans.* Clinically it is used as a chest rub in respiratory problems, and as part of a mixture in treating both vaginal and bladder infections. It is non-irritating, non-toxic and is an effective liver stimulant, which helps support recovery from illness.

Eucalyptus. Eucalyptus is used widely in upper and lower respiratory infections. It is exceptional in conditions of viral and bacterial origin. When using eucalyptus, one must distinguish between the different forms. Eucalyptus purchased for two to four dollars at a drug store has limited value (it is adulterated). *Eucalyptus radiata* is an inexpensive and highly effective antiviral oil. It also works well as an expectorant. This might be used when there is loose mucus that is not easily brought up. *Eucalyptus globulus* is an expectorant and a mucolytic agent. This can be used when there is heavy mucus congestion. Eucalyptus is administered by inhalation or chest rub. It is used in bronchitis, cold, influenza and sinusitis.

Inula graveolens. This oil is used in problems of the bronchial tract. It is an immune stimulant that has a relaxing effect on the muscles of the respiratory tract. It helps reduce mucus production and inflammation. Inula is helpful in laryngitis, chronic bronchitis and asthma. Inhalation is the usual way this oil is used. Inula is rather expensive, but its effectiveness (and the small amounts required) is worth it.

Lavender. Lavender is one of the most widely used and effective of the essential oils. It is generally not used in the acute stages of bacterial infection, but can be used to boost immunity as a preventive. Lavender has been shown to be helpful against herpes simplex, or cold sores, and perhaps for genital herpes. It is a useful antiseptic with cuts or burns.

To some it may seem odd that the oil of a plant would possess such potent effects against infectious illness. Indeed, flowery names such as rosemary and lavender conjure more an image of perfume than a potent biological substance. But do not be deceived. Mother Nature has designed plants to produce substances that are helpful in protecting them against predatory and parasitic insects as well as the microbial world. It is the plant's own form of defense. These same substances have proven extremely useful in human illness. With recent advances in chemistry, scientists are beginning to unravel the mystery of why and how these plants act as such potent healers.

Application of Essential Oils

Essential oils can be used through the nose and lungs via inhalation, through the nose via drops, by mouth via drops or a liquid mixture, through the skin via rubbing, and rectally via suppository. Each has advantages in different situations. Some oils are skin irritants and are best taken other ways. Others are delivered more quickly by inhalation, such as in lung congestion. One way to accomplish this is by use of a diffusor, which vaporizes the oil so it can be breathed. Many different diffusors are available. AromaSys, Inc., of Minneapolis, Minnesota manufactures the most technologically advanced diffusor available. The cost is in line with other diffusors.

Safety of Essential Oils

The essential oils discussed in this book are generally safe when used in the recommended dosages. Various oils have the potential for toxicity when used in excess. However, most of these oils are not employed in aromatherapy. Some people experience allergic reactions to essential oils, but this is uncommon. Certain essential oils taken for extended periods may cause chronic toxicity. Consult a physician before using essences internally with small children or pregnant women. In his book *The Art of Aromatherapy,* Robert Tisserand addresses safety issue in some depth, concluding with this remark: "There is minimal risk of allergic reaction, and no risk of toxicity if essences are prescribed in the doses given for no longer than the period of time given. There is even less risk when using essences externally. . . ."[23] Anyone taking essential oils who is concerned about safety issues should read Tisserand's book.

Using Essential Oils to Prevent Infection and Boost Immunity

Essential oils can be used very effectively to *prevent* microbes from gaining a foothold and to boost immunity. There are two basic approaches. First, they can be used once or twice a week during the winter months when common infections are most probable. Second, they can be used daily when family members or co-workers have become sick with something you want to avoid. The basic approach is to use certain oils in the shower or bath when your skin is wet. The oil constituents are absorbed into the skin and transported through the blood, where they exert their immune-boosting action.

Any of the following oils or oil mixtures may be tried:

Mix one drop of savory oil in a 2 ounce bottle of tea tree oil. In the middle of your shower, rub the oil on your chest, back and legs and let stand for 10 seconds. Then simply rinse the oil off with cool water.

An alternative is to use Niaouli (or MQV) liberally as you would the above mixture. Another option is to use *Eucalyptus radiata* or lavender oil as above. If this process causes drying of the skin, you may wish to follow your shower with a body oil rub or oil of *Rosa rubiginosa.*

For more information on the use of essential oils, see:

The Art of Aromatherapy by Robert Tisserand (Rochester, Vermont: Healing Arts Press, 1977).

The Practice of Aromatherapy by Jean Valnet (Rochester, Vermont: Healing Arts Press, 1982).

Aromatherapy to Heal and Tend the Body by Robert Tisserand (Santa Fe, New Mexico: Lotus Press, 1988).

Homeopathic Medicine:
Stellar History, Brilliant Future

While many people in the West are unfamiliar with homeopathy, its use and popularity are growing worldwide. Homeopathic medicine has historically been an effective means of combating infectious disease. Dana Ullman, M.P.H., has written extensively on the use of homeopathy. In a chapter on infectious disease, published in his book *Homeopathy: Medicine for the 21st Century,* he writes, "A little known fact of history is that homeopathic medicine developed its popularity in both the United States and Europe because of its successes in treating epidemics that raged during the 19th century. Dr. Thomas L. Bradford's *The Logic of Figures,* published in 1900, compares in detail the death rates in homeopathic versus allopathic (conventional) medical hospitals and shows that the death rate per 100 patients in homeopathic hospitals was often one-half or even one-eighth that of conventional medical hospitals."[24,25]

Ullman continues, "In 1849, the homeopaths of Cincinnati claimed that in over a thousand cases of cholera only 3 percent of the patients died. To substantiate their results, they even printed in a newspaper the names and addresses of patients who died or survived. The death rate of cholera patients who used conventional medicine generally ranged from 40 to 70 percent."[26] "The success of treating yellow fever with homeopathy was so impressive that a report from the United States Government's Board of Experts discussed the value of several homeopathic medicines, despite the fact that the Board was primarily composed of conventional physicians who despised homeopathy."[27,28]

The following contemporary examples illustrate the value of homeopathy in managing bacterial disease. In the mid-1970s, an epidemic of meningitis was ravaging the children of Brazil. Amidst the epidemic, physicians in that country gave a homeopathic preparation of *Meningococcus* 10c (a homeopathic preparation of the bacterium *Neisseria meningitidis)* to 18,640 children. Those given the homeopathic preparation had significantly fewer cases of meningitis than did other children living in the same community.[29] In 1991–1992, a cholera epidemic raged through the continent of South America. Physicians at Sam Marcos University in Lima, Peru have found homeopathic medicine to be so effective in a pilot study of cholera, that they have now undertaken a large double-blind, placebo-controlled trial to further understand its role. According to a report published in the *British Homeopathic Journal,* "The easily applied treatment and readily obtained clinical results have convinced the physicians of the Cholera Health Centers."[30]

Homeopathy is also effective in a variety of viral illnesses. A remedy called *Oscillococcinum* has been used widely in France for treatment of the flu. Researchers have found that when taken within the first 48 hours of the flu it is 80 to 90 percent successful. Many viral illnesses of childhood can also be treated with homeopathy. Treatment of chickenpox with *Rhus tox* relieves itching, reduces severity and often shortens the duration of illness to only three to five days.

The value of homeopathy can be further illustrated by the following example. Kevin was a 38-year-old pharmacist and avid sportsman. One evening, while playing baseball, he slid into second base and sustained a severe cut to his leg from the spikes of an opposing player. The injury was quite deep and bled heavily. He cleaned and carefully bandaged the wound. After several days he developed swelling and redness around the injury and a fever of 103 degrees—signs of a systemic bacterial infection. Kevin consulted his physician G. William Jones, M.D., an internist who also practices homeopathic medicine. Dr. Jones initially felt the case required antibiotics. However, Kevin reminded him of his history of serious adverse reactions to most antibiotics. Instead of antibiotics, Dr. Jones prescribed *Belladonna* and *Pyrogen,* homeopathic medicines often helpful during this type of infection. Within 24 hours, the fever began to fall and the swelling around the injury decreased. After only three days, Kevin had fully recovered from what was clearly a bacterial infection resulting from a contaminated wound.

The lesson here is that homeopathy has a vital role to play in the care of bacterial, viral and parasitic illness. There obviously are still instances when antibiotics are required, but homeopathy can be an important adjunct even when antibiotics are used. By using homeopathy, one can take advantage of its ability to boost immunity and speed convalescence.

To single out remedies used in infectious illness is difficult since there are so many that might be considered in the care of a particular illness. However, a description can be given of those commonly used in a home-care setting. Descriptions include a few of the common symptoms associated with the particular remedy. Remedies that boost immunity during infection include:

Aconite. This remedy is used within the first 24 to 48 hours of an illness or fever that comes on rapidly without warning. Symptoms often come on after exposure to cold, trauma, shock or surgery. *Aconite* has been successfully used with cold, fever, influenza, sore throat and earache.

Apis mellifica. This remedy is used when there is acute pain accompanied by stinging, burning pain with swelling, such as in a sore throat. Symptoms are aggravated by heat and made better by cold water or cold air. *Apis* has been successfully used in sore throats, coughs, colds, injuries and conjunctivitis.

Arsenicum. This is often associated with burning pains. The throat, eyes, nose, ears, or stomach are commonly, but not always, affected. The patients feel cold and crave warmth. *Arsenicum* has been successfully used in colds, coughs, influenza, measles, mumps and sore throat.

Belladonna. Used in acute illness that comes on rapidly and without warning. There is often fever and acute pain. The cheeks are often red and the pupils dilated. *Belladonna* has been successfully used in sore throats, fevers, earaches, coughs, bladder infection and skin infections.

Rhus toxicodendron. This remedy is for symptoms of a painful throat that comes on after exposure to cold or wet weather. *Rhus tox* has been successfully used in sore throat, measles, mumps, chickenpox, coughs, colds, influenza and impetigo.

Mercurius. There is often severe sore throat accompanied by fever and weakness. The tongue is often swollen. There is heavy, foul perspiration, foul breath and a tendency to drool. Symptoms are worse with almost any environmental influence. *Mercurius* is often used when infections have produced pus. This may occur in sore throat, ear infection, conjunctivitis, urinary infections and boils.

Hepar Sulph. This remedy is used in earaches, sore throats, coughs, colds and skin infections. Areas of illness are extremely sensitive to touch or pressure, and to cold. Any cold exposure makes symptoms much worse. These patients often have foul breath. Their perspiration, nasal discharge and stools also have an offensive odor.

Lachesis. This remedy is commonly used in sore throats but is also used in coughs, colds, influenza and infections of the skin. With sore throats, the pain is usually worse on the left side or begins on the left side. The throat is sensitive to touch and painful if clothing is worn around the neck. A sensation of swelling in the throat is common.

This is just a brief summary of remedies used in infectious illness. For more information on homeopathic medicine, see:

> *Everybody's Guide to Homeopathic Medicine* by Stephen Cummings and Dana Ullman (Los Angeles: Jeremy P. Tarcher, 1984).

> *Discovering Homeopathy: Medicine for the 21st Century* by Dana Ullman (Berkeley, CA: North Atlantic Books, 1992).

Hands-On Healing

The laying on of hands has been a component of healing systems for centuries. Certain forms of touch stimulate the body's healing and defense mechanisms. There is evidence that hands-on treatment has an important role to play in prevention of illness as well as in treatment during illness.

Chiropractic

One of the tools of the chiropractic physician is the adjustment, or manipulation of the spine and the extremities.* Over the years, chiropractic physicians have reported success in treating a variety of conditions associated with bacterial and viral infection. Manipulation of the vertebrae has an influence on neurologic function, lymphatic drainage, blood flow and muscle tension. Recent research by Patricia C. Brennan, Ph.D., suggests that manipulation may also have a direct effect on certain aspects of immune function. Her group showed that when the thoracic spine (mid-back) was adjusted, the respiratory burst cycle of white blood cells was enhanced.[31] Manipulation is thought to stimulate immune function, in part by promoting the release of endorphins—long associated with improving immunity.

There is also a growing body of clinical evidence. In 1987, Gottfried Gutmann, M.D., a leading researcher in the field of manipulative medicine, reported on the examination and treatment of more than 1,000 infants and small children using manipulation of the vertebrae. His findings reveal that many common ear, nose, throat and bronchial disorders of childhood respond more favorably to adjustment of the vertebrae than to medication. He states, "If the indications are correctly observed, chiropractic can often bring about amazingly successful results, because the therapy is a causal one."[32]

German physician K. Lewit, writing in a textbook of manual medicine, reported that 92 percent of youthful patients with chronic tonsillitis had blockage, or misalignment, of the first cervical vertebra and the occiput (base of the skull). According to Dr. Lewit, "After removal of the blockage [by adjustment of the vertebrae], recurrence is absent."[33,34] Pediatrician U. Mohr has reported on cases of chronic tonsillitis in which tonsillectomy was planned. However, after treatment of the functional disturbances of the

---

*Many chiropractic physicians also employ the use of acupuncture, homeopathic medicine, herbal medicine, dietary therapy and lifestyle counseling. They are one of the largest groups of health professionals in the U.S. who use clinical nutrition in their practice. Unlike medical licensing exams, the chiropractic exams include testing of proficiency in nutrition.

spine using manipulation, the problem resolved and no tonsillectomy was needed.[35]

Recall the study by Drs. Wendy and Juan van Breda in which the rate of tonsillitis and otitis media was much lower in the children of chiropractors compared with the children of pediatricians. This might be attributed in part to fact that spinal manipulation was a part of the health care received by the chiropractic children.[36]

At the Department of Maternal and Child Health, Center for Clinical Studies at Northwestern College of Chiropractic, Carol J. Phillips, D.C., has reported on numerous cases of ear infections in children that have responded to manipulation of the vertebrae. In many cases, these children had received multiple doses of antibiotics followed by tubes, with little improvement. Dr. Phillips also reports that many cases of acute earaches respond quickly to manipulation.[37]

We are not saying that manipulation is the cure for infectious diseases. However, there is an aspect of manipulation that appears to stimulate resistance to disease. Manipulation also corrects mechanical blockages that occur following injuries. This form of treatment is worthy of consideration, especially when there is a history of birth trauma or injury later in childhood. The same holds true for adults, in whom ear, nose, throat and sinus problems are commonly seen after injuries.

Therapeutic Massage

Massage is another area known to promote healing. It is now being used in hospitals throughout the world to reduce stress, aid in pain control, improve circulation, promote relaxation and stimulate the release of toxins that build up in the body. There is some evidence that massage also enhances immune function. We reported in Chapter 6 on studies showing that when animals are massaged or handled in infancy, they have better-developed immune systems later in life.

Massage also stimulates movement of lymphatic fluid through the lymph vessels. This network is an important part of the immune system and the system of elimination of toxins. Lymphatic vessels have no muscles, thus the only way fluid can move is through muscle activity created by exercise, or by physically manipulating muscles through massage. Massage may enhance immunity, in part by improving lymphatic circulation.

Some massage therapists have reported that their clients are able to get over the flu, colds, tonsillitis and other disorders more quickly when massage is part of their care. Whenever you or your child become ill, you should consider providing a full-body massage or seeking the services of a massage therapist. Massage with essential oils further enhances the treatment. During times of good health, massage can be used as part of your healthy living or prevention program. The best part may be that massage is extremely enjoyable. Treat yourself!

Acupuncture

Acupuncture is another form of healing that is being used to boost immunity and improve resistance. In a 1991 issue of the *American Journal of Chinese Medicine* published by the Institute for Advanced Research in Asian Science and Medicine, it was reported that acupuncture stimulation increased some parameters of immune function, (increased beta-endorphin in peripheral blood mononuclear cells and increased T-lymphocyte proliferation to mitogen). The investigators in this study concluded their paper by stating, "Our data are consistent with the hypothesis that the immune system might be modulated by traditional acupuncture."[38]

Acupuncture is also being investigated as a means to stimulate immunity in people with AIDS and other immunosuppressive disorders. Acupuncture is generally not used a sole means of therapy during times of lowered immunity or during infection. However, it is being used concurrently with other therapies such as botanical medicine to promote enhanced immunity.

The Logical Step

We have presented substantial evidence that antibiotics are often misused and that there may be better approaches to managing *common* infections. With the growing evidence suggesting immune-building methods might better serve our health needs, it seems logical to take a new approach. This approach would involve the use of natural substances as preventives or in the early stages of illness. If this approach is unsuccessful, antibiotics can be brought in to assist the healing process. There are certain circumstances and disorders in which antibiotic therapy is the prudent choice. But even in such cases, we must include in our treatments ways to stimulate immunity and promote healing. As we stated in the introductory remarks of this book, "Antibiotics *alone* are never the answer" because they do nothing to promote immunity or healing of injured tissue. We hope that doctors will some day recognize that their treatments will be more effective when this basic philosophy is followed. In this way, we can utilize the inherent value of antibiotics more wisely, while respecting the human body.

IV

Selfcare/Wellcare

10

Common Conditions for Which Antibiotics Are Prescribed: What You Can Do

Throughout this book we describe a variety of ways in which antibiotics are misused or inappropriately applied. Many illnesses for which antibiotics are used are common complaints that can be managed with home care. Others may require antibiotics for a brief period, but in such cases home-care remedies can also be used to stimulate natural resistance and speed recovery.

Many conditions for which people seek medical care are related to allergies, viruses or inflammation and *cannot* be helped by antibiotics. On the other hand, certain bacterial infections can be serious and life-threatening and require antibiotics. It is difficult for you to know precisely the cause of you or your child's health problems—that's why there are doctors. However, as we showed in Chapter 2, doctors are not always certain of their diagnosis. In addition, doctors are inclined to use antibiotics, sometimes in spite of research that suggests antibiotics might be of little help. That's why you need to be an informed consumer of health care. You will be better able to protect you and your child's health *and* your pocketbook.

Dr. Sehnert has advocated for many years in best-selling books such as *How to be Your Own Doctor (Sometimes)* and *Selfcare/Wellcare* the concept of the "Activated Patient" in which the patient assumes an *active* role in the management of common health problems rather than the *passive* role preferred by many doctors. He has trained thousands of people over the past 20 years by following three important assumptions:

1. Ordinary people with accurate information can treat many common health problems earlier and cheaper (and sometimes more effectively) than professionals.

2. People don't need a formal medical education to be trusted to take care of themselves.

3. Knowledge about health should not be a guarded secret for doctors, nurses and health professionals, but should be shared with lay people, particularly when the information is clearly stated. This is part of medical self care.

When illness arises in your family, both you and your doctor should ask the following questions.

1. Is the problem related to bacterial infection? Was a culture done?

2. If so, what type of bacterium is present?

3. Which antibiotic will be effective against this particular bacterium?

4. If an antibiotic is required, is it best to give it immediately?

5. Is it best to give the antibiotic later and allow the immune system to do its work? What are the consequences if you wait?

6. Is it best to withhold antibiotics altogether?

7. Are there alternatives to antibiotics?

8. What are the likely consequences if you do not use antibiotics?

Ask your doctor these questions. The doctor may be reluctant or unable to answer them. However, if he gives you good reasons for proceeding with antibiotic therapy, you should follow his advice. If the doctor has not addressed the above questions or has not given you a satisfactory answer to them, you should be more cautious.

Below is a directory of common conditions for which antibiotics are prescribed and remedies that can be used at home. Whenever symptoms persist see your doctor, but remember that the

224

supportive methods listed below can also be helpful when medical care is sought.

Acne

The Nature and Cause. Acne is the most common of all skin disorders. Males are more often affected than females. It usually occurs in children, beginning at puberty and persisting through adolescence. In some individuals, acne can remain a problem to age 50 or 60. The cause is unknown, although doctors believe it is due to problems in the sebaceous glands of the skin.

The Diagnosis. Pimples usually occur over the face, back and shoulders.

Customary Treatment. Acne is usually treated with antibiotics or with Retin-A® and with a topical steroid (cortisone derivative) drug. Oral contraceptives are sometimes found to be helpful. The antibiotics most often used include erythromycin and tetracycline (Clindamycin®).

Complications. Cyst formation can be a problem. Permanent scarring may also occur, especially in severe acne. Perhaps the greatest complication is psychological.

Natural Remedies. Although certain individuals respond well to dietary manipulation, many doctors consider this approach controversial. Numerous studies have shown zinc to be one of the most important nutrients used in acne treatment. Amounts used in these studies were generally between 90 and 135 milligrams daily for one to three months (a doctor should be consulted before using this amount of zinc). In addition to zinc, the following program has produced good to excellent results in 92 percent of patients.[1,2]

1. Avoid inorganic *iron* (inactivates vitamin E).

2 Avoid *female hormones* (antagonistic to vitamin E).

3. Avoid extra *iodine* (can aggravate acne).

4. Avoid commercial soft drinks with brominated vegetable oil (can make acne worse).

5. Avoid over 1 glass of *milk* daily (hormones in the milk can aggravate acne).

6. Avoid excess *vitamin B₁₂* (can produce or aggravate acne).

7. *Vitamin A* (water-soluble) 50,000 IU twice daily before meals. Do not use this amount without the advice of a physician.

8. *Vitamin E* 400 IU twice daily before meals.

9. *Pyridoxine* (B₆) 50 mg once or twice daily for premenstrual and menstrual acne.

10. *Benzoyl peroxide* 5 percent gel applied at night after washing gently with nonmedicated soap. Some Australian dermatologists use 5 percent tea tree oil gel with better success.

11. Well-balanced diet, low in *fat* and *sugars*.

Essential plant oils are sometimes used to care for acne. Rosewood oil or tea tree oil dabbed onto emerging blemishes can be very effective. The scars of acne (and scars due to other causes) can be effectively treated using the daily topical application of *Rosa rubiginosa* and helichrysum.* With several month's use, the results can sometimes be astonishing.

Bladder Infection (Cystitis)

The Nature and Cause. Bladder infections, or urinary tract infections, (UTI) affect roughly 25 million American women each year. They are rare in men until after age forty. Girls under the age of two are commonly affected because of improper wiping after a bowel movement, which forces fecal bacteria into the urethra. Seventy percent of infections are caused by the common intestinal bacterium *E. coli.* UTIs appear to be more common among sexually active women, in part because *E. coli* is spread from the rectum to the urethra during intercourse. In some individuals UTIs occur repeatedly, suggesting an underlying problem such as poor nutrition or improper hygienic practices.

---

*Information on the use of essential oils was provided with the assistance of Kurt Schnaubelt, Ph.D., Pacific Institute of Aromatherapy, P.O. Box 6723, San Rafael, California 94903 (415) 479-9121.

Bladder infections can also occur following antibiotic treatment for an upper respiratory tract infection[3] or from use of spermicidal preparations such as those containing nonoxynol-9 (e.g. Semicide® Vaginal Contraceptive Inserts and Today® Vaginal Contraceptive Sponges).

Roughly 500,000 women in America who have symptoms of urinary tract infection may actually suffer from a condition known as interstitial cystitis (IC)—not responsive to antibiotics or even many natural treatments, though food allergy is often found to be a contributor. The only way to determine if IC is present is by cystoscopy, or viewing the inside of the bladder with a fiber optic probe.

The Diagnosis. The most common symptom is burning pain on urination. Thirty percent of those with bladder infection have no symptoms. Sometimes cloudy, foul-smelling or dark urine will be present. The presence of nitrates in the urine suggests but does not confirm the presence of bacteria. The most accurate laboratory test is a urine culture for bacteria.

Customary Treatment. Trimethoprim-sulfamethoxazole and ampicillin are among the antibacterials commonly used to treat UTIs. The antibiotics chloromycetin and tetracycline (for penicillin-allergic patients) are also used. People with recurrent UTIs often harbor bacteria resistant to many antibiotics. Antibiotic treatment of UTIs in women commonly triggers a vaginal yeast infection (see "vaginitis").

Complications. Although they can be quite painful, UTIs are rarely serious except in pregnant women. Occasionally the infection will spread to the kidneys, producing back pain and fever. In men over 40, UTIs often indicate the presence of prostatitis, or inflammation of the prostate.

Natural Remedies. Cranberry juice remains one of the most effective means of combating UTIs. Researchers reporting in the *New England Journal of Medicine* found that the juice of cranberries and blueberries (consumed by mouth) prevented the attachment of bladder-infecting *E. coli* to body cells. According to Harvard professor Dr. Edwin Kass, "Cranberry juice can eliminate bacteria even in those whose bladder infections have been resistant to previous antibiotic therapy."[4] Substances in cranberry juice inhibit attachment of bacteria to the wall of the bladder or urethra and work as a preventive and treatment. There is one draw-back, however; most brands of commercial cranberry juice contain only 10 percent cranberry juice, which is mixed with sugars that counteract the beneficial components of the cranberry.

Raw, flash pasteurized (low heat method) cranberry juice is available and should be the form used to care for UTIs. Walnut Acres (Penns Creek, PA, 17862, 800-433-3998) markets a juice that is 100 percent pure cranberry. A supplement is also available, Crangel, that contains 3,000 mg of concentrated cranberry juice powder—the equivalent of 8 ounces of *pure* cranberry juice (Nutrition Dynamics, Maple Plain, MN 55359, 800-444-9998). Vitamin C and bioflavonoids work synergistically to enhance the effectiveness of cranberry or blueberry juice.

Also helpful in UTIs: 3,000–8,000 milligrams of vitamin C daily; acidophilus; 5,000 IU vitamin A; 50,000 IU beta-carotene; *Cantharis,* a homeopathic medicine, 3x daily; drink extra fluid; good hygiene; frequent urination; urinate after intercourse; avoid the use of spermicides.

Oral supplementation with acidophilus in addition to use of acidophilus in a vaginal douche (two capsule of acidophilus in 4 ounces of warm water) can be very helpful in managing bladder infections. In one study, acidophilus suppositories were used intravaginally once per week for one year in women who suffered from frequent bladder infections. There was a dramatic 78 percent reduction in infections.[5] Any time antibiotics are taken for a bladder infection, acidophilus by mouth should be used concurrently.

Essential plant oils are extremely effective in controlling bladder infections. They are especially helpful in reducing the acute pain. Take 2 drops of tea tree oil by mouth every 15 minutes for the first 6 to 8 hours of symptoms. After that, gradually extend the time between doses. For chronic bladder infections, combine 5 parts thyme oil with 95 parts tea tree oil: take 2 drops of this mixture 4 times a day. This can safely be used for several months if needed. In one doctor's experience, this regimen has been effective in more than 90 percent of simple bladder infections.[6] Essential oils can be obtained from Original Swiss Aromatics (P.O. Box 6842, San Rafael, CA 94903, 415-459-3998) or from a specialty herb store. Make sure the oils are listed as "genuine and authentic" as there is a vast difference in the purity of essential oils sold to consumers.

Bronchitis

The Nature and Cause. The bronchi are the large breathing tubes that lead from the trachea to the lungs. Bronchitis can be due to bacterial, fungal or viral infection, or allergy. Exposure to particulates and pollutants can also contribute to irritation of the airway. Both food allergy and airborne allergy can lead to excessive mucus buildup in the respiratory tract. Symptoms usually include any deep, chesty cough where there is no involvement of the actual lung tissue. Pneumonia, on the other hand, describes a condition where fluid accumulates in alveoli, or tiny air sacs, in the lungs. Pneumonia should be treated by your doctor.

The Diagnosis. The doctor examines the lungs using a stethoscope, observing for various respiratory sounds. Chest x-rays may be taken to determine the severity of lung involvement. Sputum (coughed-up phlegm) cultures are sometimes done to determine whether bacteria or viruses are present. A blood test called a "CBC with a differential" will probably be done. A CBC with differential includes a count of the total number of red and white blood cells in addition to their size and type. It also includes a test for hemoglobin, which gives some indication of iron status (though there are better tests for this).

Customary Treatment. Antibiotics used in bronchitis believed due to bacteria usually include tetracycline, ampicillin or trimethoprim.

Complications. Complications of bronchitis, especially in older individuals or children can be serious. In chronic bronchitis, respiratory failure, pneumonia and cardiovascular problems can occur. If congestion moves into the lung tissue pneumonia can develop.

Natural Remedies. Vitamin A deficiency can predispose children to infections of the respiratory tract. In a study of children with measles complicated by pneumonia, those given vitamin A recovered twice as quickly, had less croup and spent fewer days in the hospital. In those treated with vitamin A, the risk of serious complications or death was reduced by 49 percent.[7] In another study, vitamin A supplementation caused a significant reduction in respiratory tract complaints.[8]

Vitamin C should be taken, 6,000 to 10,000 mg per day, along with 10,000 IU of vitamin A, 100,000 IU of beta-carotene, and 25 mg of zinc.

Essential oils can be very helpful when bronchitis strikes. For bronchitis that is accompanied by heavy mucus and unproductive cough, use *Rosemary verbinone* and *Inula graveolens* in equal portions (anise seed oil can be added for extra benefit). This can be inhaled through a diffusor four times per day and rubbed on the chest four times per day.

For bronchitis not associated with heavy mucus, use *Eucalyptus radiata* and Niaouli. This can be rubbed on the chest and inhaled.

The Common Cold

The Nature and Cause. The common cold is the most common infection of humans and is due to viruses. Bacteria do *not* cause this illness. Emotional status, stress, nutritional status and other factors all affect susceptibility to the common cold. Colds are more serious among the elderly. In one study of people over 65, cold symptoms persisted from two to 46 days, with a period of "genuine symptoms" for 18 days.[9]

Cold viruses do not spread as easily among family members as influenza viruses, but it is still important to wash your hands and follow the guidelines presented in Chapter 6.

The Diagnosis. The diagnosis is usually made based on symptoms that include runny nose, watery eyes, nasal congestion, scratchy throat, headache, chills and sometimes low fever (101°F). Laboratory tests for viruses are occasionally done to rule out more serious infection. When acute respiratory symptoms are present, doctors must rule out pneumonia, influenza and other diseases. The blood test CBC with a differential may be helpful.

Customary Treatment. There is no successful medical *treatment* for the common cold, although symptomatic treatments are available. A recent article published in *Medical World News* reveals that many methods commonly used to treat colds may be counterproductive. Antihistamines have been shown to have minimal benefit. Researchers investigating aspirin, ibuprofen and acetaminophen found that all produced "a significant increase in nasal stuffiness." Another negative report was that aspirin and acetaminophen suppressed immune function. Cold specialists agree that taking multiple-agent cold preparations is ill-advised. It is better to take one or two with a narrow spectrum of action that matches your symptoms.[10]

In 1983, more than 3 million people sought medical care for the common cold or flu. Of these, 51 percent were *needlessly* given antibiotics. Antibiotics do nothing for the common cold.[11] According to the text *Infections: Recognition, Understanding and Treatment,* "Antibiotics are not indicated even when the patient is febrile [feverish]. Many controlled prospective studies have shown that therapy with penicillin, tetracycline, or a macrolide neither influences the course of the disease nor diminishes the frequency of bacterial superinfection either in young children, or when fever is present."[12]

Complications. Serious complications of the cold usually occur only in immune-suppressed individuals. In generally healthy children, the most common complication is middle ear inflammation, or otitis media. Roughly 50 percent of all earaches are preceded by an upper respiratory problem such as a cold. Bronchitis or sinus infection may sometimes follow. Pneumonia is another complication of the cold that, although uncommon, can be serious. This complication is more common among the elderly.

Doctors often justify their use of antibiotic treatment of colds by their wish to prevent secondary bacterial infection. However, use of antibiotics to treat colds often gives rise to *super-infections,* such as pneumonia, by antibiotic-resistant bacteria.

Natural Remedies. There are a number of natural remedies that seem to shorten the duration and severity of the common cold or flu. Zinc lozenges or zinc and vitamin C lozenges can reduce the symptoms of colds.[13]

High doses of vitamin C, 1 gram per hour (especially when given intravenously) can stop a cold in hours to days. Cold expert Dr. Eliot C. Dick was recently surprised when his study of the common cold showed that use of vitamin C resulted in "symptoms and signs that were much, much milder" than their counterparts receiving placebo.[14]

Another product that has met with good clinical success in terminating common cold symptoms is Perque 1, an amino acid capsule that has free-radical quenching properties (Seraphim, Inc.)

Essential plant oils can be used to dramatically speed recovery from the common cold. *Eucalyptus radiata* can be inhaled and rubbed on the chest several times a day. If there is fever and joint pain, take one or two drops of *Ravensare aromatica* by mouth every 4 hours or so. This oil often gives a tremendous burst of energy, especially when used in the early stages of a cold.

Earaches

The Nature and Cause. Earache, or otitis media, is the most common condition for which parents bring their children to the doctor. Sensitivity (or allergy) to food or airborne substances is a common contributor to earaches. Dairy products such as milk and cheese are common culprits. Infection by the bacteria *Haemophilus influenzae* or *Streptococcus pneumoniae* accounts for the middle ear problems of some children. Infection by viruses occurs in some children, especially those who have been unresponsive to antibiotic treatment. This is often accompanied by yeast/fungal infections as an aftermath of broad-spectrum therapy.

Dietary and nutritional factors also play a role in the development of earaches. Zinc and vitamin A deficiency lead to changes in the middle ear cells and contribute to the buildup of fluid. Consumption of the wrong types of dietary fats sets the stage for inflammation in the middle ear.

The Diagnosis. Diagnosis is based primarily on examination of the eardrum using an otoscope. Tympanometry (electronic monitoring of the eardrum) is more reliable and is also commonly used. Physical symptoms are considered but are not a consistent indicator of the middle ear condition. Cultures of middle ear fluid are the best way to be certain of whether an inflamed middle ear contains bacteria. However, cultures are rarely done because an incision in the eardrum is required, and most doctor's offices are not set up to do this. The blood test CBC with a differential may be done, but it does not indicate anything about middle ear status. Blood tests are of little value in middle ear problems.

In one study of almost 4,000 children involving doctors from nine countries, doctors were certain of their diagnosis of otitis media in only 58 percent of children under one year of age.[15] With this great a margin of error, the possibility of prescribing antibiotics to a child with no bacteria in the middle ear is quite high.

Customary Treatment. Antibiotic therapy is the most common form of treatment for otitis media. Roughly 42 percent of all antibiotics prescribed to children are prescribed for otitis media. Therapy usually is recommended for 10 days. Recent studies have shown that antibiotics may not be effective for many children with otitis media. An article published in the *Journal of the American Medical Association* in 1991 showed that children who received amoxicillin for chronic earaches suffered two to six times the rate of recurrent ear problems. Similar results were reported for Pediazole® and cefaclor.[16] In addition, the appropriateness of the 10-day course of therapy has been questioned. Antibiotic schedules of two, three, five and seven days have yielded results comparable to the typical 10-day course.[17,18,19,20,21]

Experts point out that 30 to 50 percent of painful middle ears contain no bacteria.[22] Antibiotics would be of little use in such children. Moreover, up to 70 percent of children who have been unresponsive to antibiotic therapy or surgery have no bacteria in their middle ears.[23,24]

The placement of tubes in the eardrums of children with recurring earaches is the most common surgical procedure performed on children. A patient recently seen by Dr. Sehnert had had six sets of tubes placed in his ears despite little evidence of any benefit. While many doctors recommend this procedure, controversy surrounds its use. In one study, children with two infected ears were treated by placing a tube in one ear and leaving the other ear to chance. The two ears were then compared over a five-year period. In the first couple of months, the ear with the tube did slightly better. However, beyond six months there was no difference in the two ears with regard to fluid and rate of recurrent infections. In fact, there was slightly more eardrum scarring and hearing loss in the ear in which the tube had been placed.[25] Similar findings were reported in a

1990 issue of the *Pediatric Infectious Disease Journal.*[26,27]

Complications. Eardrum scarring, cholesteatoma, etc., are among the physical complications associated with otitis media. Hearing loss, intellectual impairment and delays in language development can occur when middle ear problems are long-standing.

Meningitis and mastoiditis are the most serious complications of otitis media. They usually require antibiotic or surgical treatment.

Natural Remedies. Eardrops made from a tincture of *Plantago major* can be placed in each painful ear provided there is no drainage (or tube). This herb can be obtained from an herb store or health food store. *Plantago major* can provide significant symptomatic relief.

According to ear, nose and throat specialist Dr. Fred Pullen of Miami, Florida, "Seventy-five percent [of children with recurrent ear problems] respond by the simple procedure of taking away milk products."[28] It is very important to consider food intolerance as a possible contributor, especially if there is a history of antibiotic use or a family history of allergy.

Children with earaches can usually benefit from an acidophilus supplement. Infants should use a bifidus supplement, but acidophilus is acceptable. Vitamin C, 1,000 mg three times a day, can be given to children with earaches. Zinc, 15 mg a day can also be helpful, but don't continue for more than a few weeks without a doctors advice. Avoid all processed food and refined sugar.

Homeopathic remedies can be quite helpful during acute earaches. *Pulsatilla* is often used when an earache follows a cold. There is often a greenish discharge from the nose. The child is gentle, weepy, sensitive and wants to be held all the time. *Chamomilla* is also used in acute earaches when the child is irritable and cranky and does not want to be held. This remedy is also helpful for teething discomfort. *Belladonna* is a homeopathic remedy that is used in acute earaches that come on rapidly with great pain. There is usually a fever with flushed cheeks and a hot face.

Essential plant oils can be used effectively as eardrops. Mix 5 parts lavender oil in 95 parts flax oil, or 5 parts clary sage oil in flax oil. Drop three drops in each ear where you do not see drainage. *Inula graveolens* can be rubbed onto the skin around the painful ear several times a day.

There are many, many factors that affect middle ear problems in children. The causes and practical solutions are discussed in depth in the book *Childhood Ear Infections: What Every Parent and Physician Should Know About Prevention, Home Care and Alternative Treatment,* by Dr. Schmidt (North Atlantic Books, Berkeley, CA 1990).

Fever

The Nature and Cause. Fever is the response of the body to invasion by an infectious agent. It is a beneficial sign that the body is mounting resistance. Fever is not generally a cause for concern unless:[29]

- It persists for more than three days.
- It occurs in a child under 3 months of age.
- It is associated with vomiting, listlessness or irritability.
- It is associated with neck stiffness or difficulty breathing.
- Your child is making twitching movements.

Fever can be caused by viral, bacterial, yeast/fungal or parasitic infection. The degree of fever gives little indication of the severity of the child's condition (unless a high fever of 105°+ is associated with poisoning or encephalitis). A low-grade fever with few or no symptoms gives little cause for concern.

The Diagnosis. The diagnosis is made by thermometer. The thermometer is taken orally, rectally or in the armpit. It is nearly impossible to determine the degree of fever by touching the forehead, face or other body part.

Customary Treatment. Acetaminophen (found in Tylenol®), aspirin and antibiotics are commonly used to control fever. There is a growing number of doctors who believe that fever should *not* be treated or suppressed. In one study, children with chickenpox who were given acetaminophen for the fever and discomfort recovered more slowly than did those not given acetaminophen. The author of this study, Dr. Timothy Doran, comments, "We should be advising parents to treat the child and not the thermometer. If there's a fever, and they [the child] are not uncomfortable with it, there is no reason to give it [acetaminophen]."[30]

The use of aspirin in any viral illness is ill-advised because of the likelihood of children developing Reye's Syndrome, an often-fatal inflammation of the brain. In addition, aspirin can block the body's own inflammation-fighting machinery.

The wisdom of giving antibiotics for fever has also been seriously questioned. Dr. David M. Jaffe studied the course of high fever in 955 children under 3 who were treated at hospital emergency rooms. He wondered if antibiotics should be given routinely in such cases. One half of the children were given amoxicillin while the other half received a placebo. Dr. Jaffe found that there was virtually *no difference in fever outcome* in antibiotic-treated children when compared with those given the placebo. Only a few children, who were later found to have bacterial infection, responded to amoxicillin. Dr. Jaffe concluded that antibiotics are "not advisable" for most children with high fever.[31]

Complications. Febrile convulsions can occur with high fever. These are frightening to parents, but generally result in no permanent harm. If your child experiences febrile convulsions, check with your doctor just to be safe. Antiseizure medication used to be given to children who develop febrile seizures, but this has been found to be unnecessary and harmful. Complications can occur if a fever is associated with conditions such as severe measles or pneumonia.

Natural Remedies. Though it is best not to suppress most fevers, we recognize that some parents will become uncomfortable when a fever rises too high or their child feels ill. For this reason, we have recommended a few natural fever-controlling remedies.

Essential plant oils that help with the pain and discomfort associated with fever include German chamomile oil or tea tree oil. One drop of either oil can be added to hot water and consumed every three hours. Acidophilus mixed in water is also helpful in some cases of fever.

A mixture sometimes used to aid the body during times of fever consists of a tea made from 2 parts bonset, 2 parts yarrow and 1 part echinacea. The tea can be consumed hot every two hours.[32]

Influenza (The Flu)

Nature and Cause. The common cold is sometimes compared to a "drippy faucet," while the flu is likened to Niagara Falls. The flu is caused by a virus different from that of the common cold. The illness is highly contagious and comes on suddenly. The time from exposure to the onset of symptoms is only two to three days. Symptoms include fever (two to four days), muscle aches, chills, headache, loss of appetite, malaise and lethargy. Sneezing and coughing can occur but are not as common as with colds. Influenza (along with pneumonia, a common complication of influenza) is responsible for more bed disability days than any other cause.

The Diagnosis. The diagnosis is made primarily based on the symptoms listed above.

Customary Treatment. There is no medical treatment for influenza. Antibiotics are sometimes used to treat bacterial complications should they occur. However, if antibiotics are used too early, they can undermine the healing process. Vaccination against the flu is often recommended for the elderly.

Complications. Influenza can result in serious complications in some population groups, especially the elderly. Pneumonia is the most serious of the complications. In the early 20th century, millions of Americans died as a result of a particularly virulent influenza epidemic.

Natural Remedies. Vitamin C (mineral ascorbate or esterfied ascorbate) 1,000 milligrams per hour should be taken with the first signs of the flu and continued until symptoms subside. Rest is essential. Stay in bed for a few days. Drink plenty of fluids. You may wish to soak in a hot bath containing oil of lavender and clary sage. As with the common cold, the product Perque 1, two tablets or more (up to five have been prescribed and found to be helpful) three times daily, have a beneficial result.

The essential oil *Eucalyptus radiata* can be rubbed on the chest and inhaled several times a day. One drop of *Ravensare aromatica* can be taken occasionally by mouth to improve energy.

The homeopathic remedy *Oscilococcinum* can be taken several times a day by mouth and is best taken within the first 48 hours of the onset of symptoms. This remedy is widely used in Europe. It is usually available at health food stores.

Intestinal Infections with Diarrhea

The Nature and Cause. Intestinal infection can occur from bacteria, viruses, fungi, yeast or parasites. These infections can be contracted from food, water, siblings, playmates, foreign travel or day care. The latter is probably one of the most common sources of infections among preschool children. Infection by the bacteria *Salmonella* and *Campylobacter* is a common form of food poisoning.

The Diagnosis. The diagnosis can only be accurately made by examining a stool specimen or by intestinal biopsy (not usually done).

Customary Treatment. Once the diagnosis is made, the proper antimicrobial substance can be chosen. Antibiotics are used when bacteria such as *Salmonella* are found. Antiparasitic drugs are used when parasites such as *Giardia lamblia* are identified. When viruses are found, there is little that conventional medicine has to offer. In all of the above cases, there are natural remedies that can be used that have a broad spectrum of action. In many cases, these remedies are superior to the commonly used drugs. When the infection is severe, drugs must be used. However, the natural remedies can be used concurrently to enhance results and minimize side effects.

Complications. The complications from intestinal infection are generally not severe, but are too numerous to mention in detail. The most common complication is disruption of digestion and absorption of nutrients. Another is disruption of the normal balance of bacteria that reside in the gut. Development of food allergies frequently accompanies intestinal infection, especially in children. Intolerance to cow's milk products is common following any kind of intestinal infection.

If diarrhea persists for more than one week, it can affect nutrient status and immune function. When diarrhea persists for several weeks, these effects can be serious.

Natural Remedies. *Lactobacillus acidophilus* and *Bifidobacterium bifidus* can be taken by mouth to restore normal balance and compete with and kill many harmful organisms. The dosage is usually ½ teaspoon in a glass of warm water three times per day for children and two to three capsules (one to two teaspoons powder) three times daily for adults. Acidophilus or bifidus made by Ethical Nutrients or by UAS Laboratory are of high quality.

Inner Strength® (also known as Probioplex®) is a food supplement that can thwart the activity of up to 17 different intestinal invaders including the yeast *Candida albicans,* the bacteria *E. coli* associated with travelers diarrhea and *Shigella,* associated with dysentery. When taken with acidophilus, the activity of Inner Strength® is enhanced many-fold. One teaspoon in a glass of warm water three times per day is a common adult dose during illness. For a child, ¼ teaspoon three times daily. Inner Strength® is available from Ethical Nutrients (971 Calle Negocio, San Clemente, CA 92672, 800-692-9400).

A child with diarrhea due to any cause should be given plenty of fluids that are high in electrolytes. Dr. Leo Galland recommends giving a drink made from one part fruit juice to two parts water with a pinch of salt. This helps supply fluid, sodium, potassium and sugar. (We generally don't recommend extra sugar for children, but during prolonged diarrhea it can be life-saving.) Also, give your child a ripe, mashed banana. If the diarrhea is liquid, the juice and banana should be given every ten minutes. As the diarrhea becomes more firm, the time can be extended gradually.[33]

Post-Antibiotic Syndrome

The Nature and Cause. You'll seldom find this illness listed in any medical textbooks. Yet, many doctors are beginning to recognize that the prescribing of round after round of antibiotics to children and adults has resulted in a complex series of events that suppresses the immune system while trapping the patient in a general state of poor health. These individuals often suffer from problems ranging from skin disorders to recurrent infections, from diarrhea to depression.

The Diagnosis. The diagnosis is based in part on the history. These individuals have often suffered from a bout of otitis media, sinusitis or some upper respiratory problem (often viral) in early life that was treated with antibiotics. The condition commonly did not respond to one course of antibiotics, so another was prescribed. This pattern continued for many months or even years. Throughout this period, the true cause of the illness went unnoticed and therefore untreated. Meanwhile, the adverse effects of the antibiotic treatment itself were setting in.

Signs and symptoms fall into the following categories:

1. Intestinal (pain, bloating, flatulence, poor digestion, diarrhea, constipation).

2. Allergic (food and airborne allergies).

3. Behavioral (irritability, depression, lethargy, chronic fatigue).

4. Immunologic (susceptibility to recurrent infections).

5. Dermatologic (rashes, hives, yeast infections).

6. Respiratory (chronic cough, postnasal drainage, chronic earache).

A test called the Comprehensive Digestive Stool Analysis (CDSA) should be performed to assess the function of the digestive system and intestines, and to determine the balance of bacteria in the intestines. A stool test for parasites should also be done. Tests are also available that test for permeability of the intestine. This test helps determine if you have a "leaky gut" and why digestive problems and food intolerance may persist (Great Smokies Diagnostic Laboratory, 18A Regent Park Boulevard, Asheville, NC 28806, 800-522-4762). Tests for food intolerance or allergy are also helpful.

Customary Treatment. This condition has been given little attention in Western medicine because the syndrome is largely iatrogenic (doctor-induced). What makes it all the more difficult is that the syndrome does not fit into the neat package of signs and symptoms that doctors prefer to work with. Its falls into the category of what clinicians call a "wastebasket diagnosis," or one that is used because others have been excluded. However, the syndrome is all too real to its sufferers.

Complications. The main complications are immune suppression, digestive problems, fatigue and chronic poor health. Chronic problems falling into one or more of the six categories listed above are significant complications and must be considered in anyone who has received repeated doses of antibiotics.

Natural Remedies. This condition is not highly responsive to home care practices because it is so complex and often involves so many body systems. A health professional who is skilled at working with this should be consulted. There are a few home remedies that can be used with some success.

Lactobacillus acidophilus and *Bifidobacterium bifidus* can be taken by mouth to restore their numbers. These "good" bacteria are the first to be wiped out by antibiotic therapy. Acidophilus and Bifidus also compete with and kill many harmful organisms that might invade the intestines. The dosage is usually ½ teaspoon in a glass of warm water three times per day for children and two to three capsules (one to two teaspoons powder) three times daily for adults. Acidophilus or bifidus made by Ethical Nutrients or by UAS Laboratory are of high quality.

Inner Strength® (also known as Probioplex®) is a food supplement that can thwart the activity of up to 17 different intestinal invaders including the yeast *Candida albicans,* the bacteria *E. coli* associated with travelers diarrhea and *Shigella,* associated with dysentery. When taken with acidophilus, the activity of Inner Strength® is enhanced many-fold. One teaspoon in a glass of warm water three times per day is a common adult dose during illness. For a child, ¼ teaspoon three times daily. Inner Strength® is available from Ethical Nutrients (971 Calle Negocio, San Clemente, CA 92672, 800-692-9400).

Vitamins A, E and C, the B-vitamins, flax oil, primrose oil, beta-carotene, zinc, magnesium, and selenium are other important nutrients.

Rhinitis/Stuffy Nose

The Nature and Cause. The image of the "runny-nosed toddler" with dark circles under the eyes and thumb in the mouth is probably forever burned into the memory of most parents. It is not a serious illness, yet it alerts you to the fact that something is not quite right. For some children it can interfere with breathing and disrupt sleep. In others it can be a prelude to earaches. Rhinitis is all too common in adults as well. Rhinitis or stuffy nose is usually due to allergy or viral infection, but can be linked to nutritional deficiency.

In the winter months, furnaces recirculate millions of particles that can irritate the nasal lining. Furnaces also dry out the air inside the home, lowering humidity and drying out mucous membranes that are supposed to protect children from viruses, bacteria and allergens. Cold outdoor air can also trigger or aggravate rhinitis, but this form is usually short-lived.

The Diagnosis. Diagnosis is made based on a history of a runny or stuffy nose and evidence of nasal discharge or obstruction. Cultures for respiratory syncitial virus (RSV) or rhinoviruses are sometimes done.

Customary Treatment. Antihistamines and decongestants are commonly used to manage the symptoms. Antibiotics are also sometimes used. However, since this condition is not typically due to bacterial infection, antibiotics are of questionable value.

Complications. Earaches can follow a chronic stuffy nose. In children with lowered immunity, viral or allergy-related rhinitis can sometimes move into the lower respiratory tract.

Natural Remedies. Vitamin C has been shown to be effective at doses of 1,000 to 2,000 milligrams, and higher amounts may be needed. Beta-carotene is also helpful.

Allium cepa is a homeopathic medicine that can be given four times per day when there is sneezing associated with watery eyes and runny nose. Nasal discharge is clear, watery and irritates the skin of the upper lip. The tears are non-irritating.

The homeopathic medicine *Euphrasia* can also be given when there is nasal discharge with watery eyes. However, this medicine is used when the nasal discharge is non-irritating and the tears are highly irritating. The symptoms are the reverse of *Allium cepa.*

Nosedrops can be made from the following oils: add 0.25 percent oil of *Inula graveolens,* 2.0 percent *Calophyllum inophyllum* and 0.25 percent *Rosemary officinalis* (verbenone) into a base of hazelnut oil. Put two to three drops of this mixture into the nose 5 to 10 times each day or as needed. This mixture is very effective whether you have a dry stuffy nose or a runny nose.

Also, humidify the air in the room in which you or your child sleep as well as that of the entire house if possible. Change the furnace filter every one or two weeks.

Sinusitis

The Nature and Cause. Sinusitis, or inflammation of the sinuses, is one of the most common health problems in America, affecting an estimated 2 million people annually. It occurs more commonly in adults and less commonly among children. The maxillary sinuses, located in the cheekbones, are most often affected. The frontal sinuses in the forehead are the second most affected area in adults, but in children are not affected until after age 10.

Sinusitis can be caused by bacteria *(Streptococcus pneumoniae* or *Haemophilus influenzae),* and less commonly by viruses and fungi. Dental abscess is a cause of sinusitis in 10 to 15 percent of adult cases.[34] Allergy to food or airborne substances can lead to acute or chronic sinus congestion as can exposure to cigarette smoke. Indoor air pollutants such as mold, fungi and vapors released from building materials are believed to be a common cause of persistent sinus problems.

The Diagnosis. The diagnosis is based on symptoms that commonly include sinus pain, congestion, nasal discharge, fever and malaise that often follow an upper respiratory infection. Pain is worse from bending over. Nasal cultures are of little value. Sinus X-rays are taken if one does not respond to treatment or experiences severe symptoms and is sicker than might be expected.

Dr. Sehnert teaches patients to test their sinuses with a simple method he calls the "toe test." This consists of firmly pressing the tips of the second, third and fourth toes between your thumb and index finger. Unusual tenderness on the left foot indicates sinuses on the left of your face are likely infected. Tenderness on the right spells trouble on the right. In many cases both sides will be involved.

Customary Treatment. Most people with sinusitis are treated with ampicillin, amoxicillin, trimethoprim-sulfamethoxazole or cefaclor. In children, ampicillin or amoxicillin are usually used. Curiously, in an article published in *Primary Care,* Dr. Howard Rabinowitz states, "Uncomplicated sinusitis usually responds spontaneously without antibiotics in 80 percent of patients."[35] According to Lowell Jones, M.D., antibiotics, when used, should be closely monitored and "are not recommended for long-term treatment."[36]

Topical decongestants (nasal sprays or inhalants) should not be used for more than three or four days. If used longer, rebound congestion may occur.

Complications. Complications are uncommon but can be serious. They include periorbital cellulitis, orbital abscess, cavernous sinus thrombosis, meningitis, brain abcess, subdural empyema and frontal osteomyelitis.[37] If you have symptoms that persist or increase in severity, or a fever develops, see a physician.

Natural Remedies. The herb *Ephedra sinica* is one of the most widely used sinus remedies available. (Avoid during pregnancy.) It is often combined with the herbs *Echinacea purpurea,* ginger root and goldenseal root. In addition, 50,000 IU beta-carotene and 6,000 mg vitamin C daily may be helpful.

Inhalation: Mix the oils of *Eucalyptus radiata* and *Eucalyptus globulus* in equal parts and inhale through a diffusor or vaporizer.

Internal: One drop of rosemary oil can be placed on a cotton swab. The swab can then be put through the nostril and held for *a few seconds* against the tissue deep in the nasal cavity. This gives a very strong sensation but is very helpful. Use this with adults only.

Topical: A mixture of the following oils can be rubbed on the skin over the sinuses. Add 2.5 percent oil of *Inula graveolens,* 4.0 percent *Calophyllum inophyllum* and 2.5 percent *Rosemary officinalis* (verbenone) into a base of 91 percent hazelnut oil. This can be used several times each day.

Also:

- Humidify the air in your home or office. This helps thin the mucus. Place a few drops of tea tree oil in the water to prevent the growth of mold.

- Avoid the overuse of topical decongestants (nasal sprays). They can prolong symptoms.

- Avoid airborne allergens such as cigarette smoke, pollen and animals.

- Avoid known or potential food allergens such as dairy products.

Teething in Children

The Nature and Cause. Teething is obviously a natural part of childhood that requires no medical treatment. However, conditions commonly associated with teething such as earaches, stuffy nose, coughs and colds often prompt parents to take their child to the doctor. Teething-associated problems like those above almost never require antibiotics. Yet a surprising number of doctors will treat, for example, a teething-associated middle ear problem with antibiotics. Left untreated, these types of problems usually heal with no treatment. Natural remedies can be used to make your child more comfortable without the adverse effects of antibiotics.

The Diagnosis. When you notice development of a cold, a stuffy or runny nose, or an earache, first check to see if there is irritation of your child's gum tissue or teeth that are beginning to erupt through the gums. This is especially true at six months of age with the first teeth and again at one year when the molars begin to come in. When a child cuts upper teeth, the nose is likely to run. When the child cuts lower teeth there is often a cough.

Customary Treatment. Teething is not usually treated, but as mentioned above, some doctors will treat the associated conditions with antibiotics. This is almost never necessary.

Complications. Complications from teething are rare. In some cases, a teething-associated otitis media will persist and require treatment.

Natural Remedies. When teething is associated with irritability or earache, the homeopathic medicine *Chamomilla* should be used 4 times per day until symptoms are gone or irritable behavior has stopped.

A tincture of the herb *Plantago major* can be placed on the inflamed gum tissue three to five times per day. This not only helps with teething discomfort, but also relieves ear pain associated with teething. It occasionally eliminates the pesky diaper rash that frequently accompanies teething. Tea tree oil, or *Melaleuca alternifolia,* can be rubbed on the gums several times each day as needed to help ease pain. It is also antibacterial and antiviral and may help prevent opportunistic infections that sometimes accompany teething. Use one of these applications, but not both.

Massaging the point He gu, or LI-4, located in the web between the thumb and forefinger on the back of the hand, can help relieve discomfort associated with teething.

Tonsillitis/Sore Throat

The Nature and Cause. Roughly 80 percent of sore throats are caused by viruses against which antibiotics have no effect.[38] Some sore throats are due to streptococcal bacteria. These can be helped by antibiotic treatment. Airborne allergy, food allergy, dry indoor air, polluted indoor or outdoor air, cigarette smoke and perfume can also contribute to sore throat. Cow's milk consumption is one often-overlooked contributor to chronic or acute tonsillitis.

Tonsillitis is rare in children under two. Beyond this, it can occur at any age. Sore throat is common among adults of any age. Cough and cold symptoms are less likely to accompany a bacterial sore throat than a viral sore throat.

The Diagnosis. Diagnosis is made by feeling and observing for enlarged glands on the neck just behind the angle of the jaw and by observing enlarged glands in the throat.

Throat culture is the only reliable way to determine whether a sore throat is due to strep. In a study of 222 people with sore throat, doctors believed that 50.5 percent had strep infections. However, culture results showed that only 13.5 percent were positive for strep. Most of these patients would have been given antibiotics needlessly.[39] A positive throat culture is no guarantee that strep bacteria are the cause of symptoms. Twenty percent of people in good health harbor the strep germ in their throats normally.

Customary Treatment. Several different antibiotics are used to manage sore throats. When antibiotics are used, the timing of treatment is important. When antibiotics are used in the first 48 hours of a strep throat infection, the chance of a child suffering recurrent strep infections *increases* by two to eight times. When antibiotic treatment is delayed a few days, the risk of recurrent episodes decreases. The down side of delaying treatment when there is a positive culture is that the risk of complications (although small) increases.[40]

A child with a positive throat culture should definitely receive antibiotics. However, home care methods should be used concurrently.

Complications. Rheumatic fever and kidney problems are the most common complications of sore throat due to streptococcal bacteria. However, these are rare. From 1985 to 1987, only 100 new cases of rheumatic fever were reported in the U.S. This has some doctors concerned, because this is a rather sharp increase from previous years.[41] Yet when compared to the general population, the numbers are small. Furthermore, from 33 to 50 percent of cases of rheumatic fever occur *without* sore throat symptoms.[42] In general, rheumatic fever is uncommon. This is especially true for children under age four and adults. Complications from viral sore throats are also uncommon. According to Dery, "Antibiotics effectively prevent rheumatic fever even if treatment is put off for several days—specifically the time required to obtain the results of a throat culture."[43]

If the glands become too large, they can obstruct the airway and interfere with breathing. This can be frightening to a child. In severe cases, it can be life-threatening. In such instances, immediate medical attention is required.

Natural Remedies. Homeopathic *Belladonna* can be given in the first 24 hours of a sore throat that has come on rapidly, especially if accompanied by fever and flushed skin. *Apis mellifica* or *Mercurius* are other commonly used remedies for sore throat.

Essential plant oils can be used both in the case of viral sore throat and bacterial tonsillitis. When you feel a sore throat coming on, take one drop of the essential oil *Cypress*. When symptoms return (10 to 20 minutes), take another drop. When symptoms return (one to two hours), take another drop. When symptoms return, take another drop. Gradually, the interval between symptoms grows larger until the pain is gone. You have averted the sore throat. You can take cypress as often as needed to relieve symptoms.

For more severe forms of sore throat that have progressed, the following oils can be used. *One* drop of savory, oregano *or* thyme oil can be placed on a charcoal tablet (available at health food stores). One tablet can be chewed or dissolved slowly in the mouth three to four times a day. An alternative is the following: Make a mixture of

247

20 drops savory oil, 20 drops thyme oil and five drops clove oil. Place one drop of this mixture on a charcoal tablet and let dissolve slowly in the mouth. Repeat three or four times a day.

These remedies should not be the only method used to treat a streptococcal sore throat. They can be very valuable in viral sore throats and to help relieve some of the discomfort associated with a bacterial sore throat (even when antibiotics are used).

Vaginitis (Yeast Infection)

The Nature and Cause. Though there are more than 20 known causes, vaginitis commonly results from an infection of the vagina by yeast, usually *Candida albicans.* It is not usually treated with antibiotics; however, it is often *caused* by antibiotic treatment, which is why we've included it here. Broad-spectrum antibiotics indiscriminately kill normal vaginal bacteria that usually keep yeast under control. Vaginal bacteria also help keep the vagina acidic, which prevents the growth of yeast. With no competition, the yeast grow unchecked.

Vaginitis can also be brought on by pregnancy, use of birth control pills, diabetes, stress, high-sugar diet, excessive or frequent douching, use of synthetic undergarments, and use of spermicides (such as those containing nonoxynol-9) or cortisone. *The most common cause of susceptibility to vaginal infection is a change in the acidity of the vagina.*

The Diagnosis. Symptoms include excessive vaginal discharge, which may smell bad and cause itching. Frequent urination and painful intercourse are common. Diagnosis is best made by a wet smear to determine which organism is present. Sometimes more than one organism is present.

Customary Treatment. Flagyl® is commonly used to treat *Trichomonas* vaginitis. Nystatin®, ketoconazole (Nizoral®) or fluconazole (Diflucan®) are used to treat *Candida* vaginitis. Though effective, long-term use of Flagyl® or ketoconazole should be avoided because of the risk of liver damage. Ironically, Flagyl® can *cause* yeast infections because it alters the acidity of the vagina.

Complications. Vaginitis is rarely serious. The greatest problem occurs when more serious causes of vaginal discharge have been ignored, such as gonorrhea or cancer. Vaginal infections can be passed from mother to child during birth. Children born to a mother with vaginal candidiasis develop oral thrush, a fungal infection of the mouth characterized by white patches or coating in the mouth and on the tongue.

Natural Medicine. While certain infections sometimes require specific treatments, general suggestions can be made that will create a better environment for healing.

Douche with unsweetened yogurt twice each day. Make sure the yogurt has not been pasteurized. Better yet, mix up a solution of acidophilus in milk, let it stand twenty minutes, and douche twice each day. It is also important to take acidophilus by mouth each day to help balance the flora of the intestinal tract. This has a significant impact on the flora of the vagina. In a recent study, women prone to recurrent vaginal infections who ate an eight-ounce carton of *unpasteurized* yogurt daily, suffered a dramatic decrease in symptoms. When they went off yogurt, the symptoms returned.[44] Many forms of yogurt do not contain viable forms of acidophilus. Acidophilus taken by mouth (provided the supplement is of good quality) is a very favorable option.

Also helpful for vaginitis is 1,000 mg vitamin C three times daily, 15 mg zinc, 300 mg magnesium, 10,000 IU vitamin A, 50,000 IU beta-carotene and 400 IU vitamin E.

Essential oils can be applied as follows:

Make a mixture of 50 drops tea tree oil *(Melaleuca alternifolia)*, 10 drops *Thymus vulgaris* (CT thymol) and 60 drops of hazelnut oil. Soak a tampon in this mixture and insert into the vagina and leave for several hours. This can be repeated three times per day.

A mixture that has mucolytic action can be made from two drops rosemary, two drops helichrysum and 60 drops hazelnut. This also can be used with a vaginal suppository. For best results, alternate the tea tree oil suppository with the rosemary suppository.

In General

In addition to the specific recommendations above, the following general strategies are often helpful.

1. Get extra rest.

2. Drink plenty of fluids.

3. Eat light if that is what your body feels.

4. Eliminate all dairy products.

5. Eliminate all sugar and processed foods.

6. Avoid cola beverages and other soda pop.

7. Avoid illicit or recreational drugs.

8. If you are on medication, especially cortisone or antibiotics, see your doctor to make sure it is necessary. These drugs commonly aggravate health problems. They should be used only when essential.

9. Incorporate laughter and humor into your healing arsenal.

Remember, we usually succumb to infection for a reason. Use of antibiotics alone rarely addresses the underlying reason one becomes ill. The above home-care remedies can often be used with great success when you become ill. Remember also to evaluate your diet, lifestyle, emotional state, stress levels and other factors discussed previously. If symptoms persist, see your doctor.

---

1. The following herbs should be avoided during pregnancy: ginseng, ephedra, goldenseal, thyme, yarrow, savory, rosemary, oregano.

2. Some dairy-sensitive individuals may react to Probioplex® or Inner Strength®. If you are dairy-sensitive, begin with very small doses or see your doctor before using.

11

50 (or so) Ways to Boost Immunity and Avoid Antibiotics

This chapter is designed to show at a glance things that influence infection-susceptibility *and* improve well-being. While no one can guarantee that you will not succumb to infection by following this advice, it is probable that you will increase your resistance. Each of the items below has been discussed in previous chapters. For more information on items of interest, please refer to the index.

Lists of "dos" and "don'ts" often seem like admonishments. They may seem reminiscent of an authority figure depriving you of free choice. That is not the intent here. As you read the points below, keep in mind that the key is to invigorate your life with fun, enthusiasm, joy, laughter and good health. Good health should never be boring. It should be vibrant. You can follow the suggestions below and still satisfy your palate, take risks, stimulate your mind, experience beauty, and have a good time. The key is common sense, balance, moderation, compassion and listening to your body.

Mood, Mind and Emotions

- Work at becoming more of an optimist. Optimists have healthier immune systems, suffer from fewer infections and are not as adversely affected by stressful life events. They in fact experience fewer negative events. Pessimism is reversible. Learn how to be an optimist. See *Learned Optimism* by Martin Seligman, Ph.D.

- Guard against cynicism and hostility. If you find yourself reacting to events with hostility, stop yourself, take some deep breaths and feel how your body is responding. Death rates in people who are hostile, cynical or suspicious are four to seven times higher than in people who are not.

- Express your feelings and emotions. Suppressed anger, sadness, grief or other emotions can lead to suppressed immunity. We all experience anger and sadness and need to express it in healthy ways. Suppressed anger has been associated with more frequent illness.

- Take control. If you are in a situation that seems outside your control, find little things over which you can exert control. A sense of control seems to help our immune systems function more efficiently.

- Be willing to ask for and accept support from friends and loved ones.

- Find a sense of meaning and purpose in your relationships, work and daily activities.

- Learn to say "no" (when you need to) when others ask for your help or services. While service and giving are important parts of a healthy life, being unable to assert yourself and claim your needs is not.

- Keep a daily journal of your *feelings,* especially during important life events. It gives the immune system a boost that can be verified as long as six weeks after the journal-keeping has been discontinued.

- Take classes in relaxation. Self-relaxation techniques have been shown to boost immunity, relieve pain and improve life in general.

- Take life less seriously. As Dr. Wayne Dyer says, "Act as though what we do really matters, but realize that it does not."

- If you are depressed, seek help from a professional. Seek out people you trust. Get moderate exercise. People suffering from depression have weakened immune systems and are more susceptible to infection.

- Laugh as much as you can. Attend funny movies, read funny stories, socialize with funny people and try to see the humorous things in life.

- Become more idealistic. Realists often have a more accurate view of the world but are also more apt to be depressed, which may lead to sluggish immunity.

- When stressful life events strike, take extra time, do relaxation exercises, write in a journal, discuss your feelings with someone you trust, stay away from junk food, take extra vitamins. During high-stress periods, we are vulnerable. The extra effort spent caring for yourself will pay off.

- Rate your health high. Begin to view yourself as healthy. Those who do actually live longer and feel better.

- Take control of your health. Do not rely on doctors. When you use doctors, try to form a health partnership. Find a doctor whose philosophy of care is similar to your own. You will be more likely to trust his/her advice and follow through with recommendations. In such a relationship, doctors are less likely to respond negatively to your questions.

Lifestyle

- Get regular exercise, even if it's only walking for 30 minutes each day. Remember, kids need exercise, too. Those who exercise moderately are more resistant to infection. Make sure the exercise is fun. Do it with a friend if at all possible. Heavy exercisers can be *more* susceptible to infection. If you are a heavy exerciser who gets ill frequently, modify your workouts.

- Partake of a weekly or biweekly sauna (especially during the high-risk winter months). It helps cleanse the body of waste products and impurities and can cut the incidence of infection. If you have heart disease, are pregnant or have circulatory problems, see your doctor before proceeding.

- Get more touch in your life. Treat yourself to a weekly therapeutic massage. Touch your spouse more often. Touch and hug your kids throughout the day. Babies especially love touch.

- Get adequate sunlight, especially if you live in a northern climate, during winter, or if you work indoors under artificial lights. Get outside on sunny winter days. Sun exposure on your hands and face is often enough, but full body is better. Avoid excessive sun exposure during summertime.

- If you smoke, give it up. If there is a smoker in your home, encourage them to quit. Smokers and those who live with smokers get more respiratory infections.

- If you are a workaholic, STOP! Take time to find out what drives the working obsession. Smell the flowers.

- Limit TV viewing hours. It contributes to a more sedentary life, obesity and poor nutrition. It takes time away from interacting with family and friends, and from introspection. It also gives the impression that the world is more violent and treacherous than it really is.

- Designate a "quiet room" in the house—especially if you have children. This is a room that allows you to escape from the stressful noise and chatter. The room should contain no TV or radio and should be off limits to others while you are inside. Try arranging quiet time for your kids as well.

- During the winter months, use essential oils daily on your skin or in the bath. The active constituents in these oils boost immune function and help prevent against infectious illness.

- Pray or meditate each day.

- Look at the health of your parents and siblings. If they are prone to certain types of illness, you may be likewise. Take preventive steps regarding lifestyle and nutrition.

- Drink alcohol only moderately, if at all.
- Avoid overuse of prescription drugs.
- Avoid use of illicit drugs.
- Get adequate sleep. Most people need 6 to 8 hours a night of uninterrupted sleep. A short nap in the afternoon is often helpful, provided it does not disrupt your evening sleep.

Diet and Nutrition

- Reduce your intake of refined sugar. Excess sugar can make the immune system sluggish.
- Reduce your intake of fat (unless it is already at or below 20 percent of your total calories). Avoid margarine and hydrogenated fats. If your triglycerides are high, work to lower them. Elevated blood fats can slow immune function.
- Increase your intake of omega-3 essential fatty acids such as those found in flax oil and fish oil (salmon, mackerel, herring, sardines, trout). You may also wish to take a perle of evening primrose oil daily, which contains the omega-6 oil gamma-linolenic acid (GLA). Those in the industrialized world often consume too little of these oils. When taking additional oils *always* take additional vitamin E (50–400 mg).
- Avoid white bread and refined flour products. They are devoid of essential nutrients including the essential fatty acids mentioned above.
- Include fiber in your diet in the form of fruits, vegetables, nuts, seeds, legumes and whole grains. These foods are also high in vitamins and minerals.
- Reduce your intake of pastries, doughnuts, french fries, chicken nuggets, candies and other foods containing "funny fats," or trans fatty acids. When these foods are consumed in excess, sluggish immunity may follow.
- Eat several smaller meals a day as opposed to three large meals a day. It is easier on all aspects of your body.

- Reduce your intake of coffee. Try the many varieties of herbal tea available.

- Reduce your intake of soft drinks. They can leach calcium and magnesium from the body.

- Follow the rhythms of your body. Eat when you're hungry, stop when you're full. Don't let the clock rule mealtime. Try mealtime without the paper, TV or radio.

- Rotate your foods to avoid boredom and monotony. Eating the same foods every day can also lead to the development of food intolerance.

- If you have a health problem, consider the possibility that the foods you consume might be part of the problem. Remember, allergies don't cause everything, but they can cause anything!

- Take a multivitamin each day with meals. It should contain no artificial colors or preservatives and should be free of wheat, corn, soy, dairy and other products likely to cause problems in sensitive people.

- Take extra vitamin C each day. 1,000 to 2,000 milligrams is a good start. Some believe higher amounts are even better.

- Take other antioxidants such as beta-carotene, vitamin E and selenium. Antioxidants are important in immune function.

- Don't be obsessive about nutrition. While a healthy, balanced diet is important to wellbeing, fretting about it may negate much of the good you've accomplished.

- Splurge on your favorite treats now and then. If you've followed the guidelines above, reward yourself. Rigidity and abstinence are not the order of the day—just moderation.

Social

- Find a community with whom you share interests. Close social ties are important to our resistance to disease.

- Cultivate interpersonal relationships. Those with more close personal ties have healthier immune systems. Those who isolate themselves are more susceptible to illness that is more severe and long-lasting.

- Play, play, play. The less we play, the more somber and serious our world becomes. Play is an absolute necessity for health and well-being.

- Plan an outing with your spouse or mate at least once a week. Plan an outing with your children where they get your undivided attention.

- Take vacations. It doesn't have to be far, just a change of scenery.

Spiritual

- Give thanks for the gifts you've been given. Say a prayer before you eat. Say a prayer before bed. Give thanks for the blessings of the day. These things are inherent in all religious traditions.

- In times of trouble, seek the solace of prayer and meditation.

- Ask for prayers from others when you become ill. Pray for yourself when ill and believe that it will be helpful.

- Recognize the sacred nature of our planet and the creatures that inhabit it.

- Whatever your religious conviction, understand the sanctity of seasonal rituals. Celebrate them and avoid the commercialization that many have come to represent.

- Avoid rigidity. Rigidity or inflexibility in one's beliefs may translate into a rigid and inflexible immune system. Remember, rigid routines were associated with increased infection duration and severity.

When You Feel Illness Approaching

- Get extra rest. Failure to get adequate rest can slow recovery and prolong illness. However, don't lie around all day. Some movement is important to recovery.

- Eliminate all junk food immediately.

- Eliminate all dairy products immediately.

- Eliminate all sugar (unless a child suffers from severe diarrhea, in which case special recommendations are in order).

- Slow down. Cut back your schedule, take time off work or leave work early. Don't be a martyr for work. Try to reduce the stress in your life at that time.

- Begin to take extra vitamin C, zinc and other nutrients.

- Begin taking the herb *Echinacea*. It is a good immune booster.

- Select the homeopathic medicine that best fits your condition. This can bring you out of an episode of illness with sometimes remarkable speed.

- Evaluate your life. Is sickness a signal that you need to slow down or take better care of yourself? Is it a sign you're not attending to some of your basic needs?

- Don't rely on doctors to solve your health problem. You are the healer. Take charge of your health. Use doctors for diagnosis and advice, but use their advice thoughtfully.

- Meditate using deep breathing.

Environment

- Limit your use of synthetic materials.

- Sauna regularly to help purge toxic compounds from your body.

- Do a periodic cleansing of your internal body using the Metabolic Clearing Therapy or some variation. Many with sluggish immune systems experience dramatic improvement following such programs. Even those who are not ill experience a heightened sense of well-being.

- If you suffer from chronic or recurrent infections, you may be toxic. Have an evaluation done by a doctor familiar with environmental medicine. Certain blood and urine tests can detect exposure to toxins you may not be aware of.

- If you work in an occupation in which chemicals are used, have regular check-ups and consider having blood and urine analysis to detect toxic exposure. It may be especially important that you do a cleanse.

- Avoid synthetic personal hygiene products.

- Take extra antioxidant nutrients including vitamins C and E, beta-carotene and selenium. Also use zinc and magnesium.

- Use liver-protecting herbs such as milk thistle seed extract.

- Drink water purified by carbon filtration and reverse osmosis, especially if you live in an area with landfills or known chemical contaminants.

- Wear protective gloves and clothing whenever working with toxic chemicals at home or at work. This includes common lawn and garden products.

Medicine Has Become Serious Business

Don't eat too much fat, stay away from the salt, exercise three times a week, don't smoke, don't drink alcohol, and on and on. Our daily lives are constantly filled with dos and don'ts. Doctors have become risk managers of our health much like attorneys are risk managers in other areas of life. It all seems like such serious business. But, good health does not have to be serious business. We don't advocate that you become a health fanatic. We don't advocate that you make every decision based on whether or not it is healthy. Nor do we suggest that health be a regular topic of conversation in your daily life. The business of good health should be a benefit of your road to personal growth and discovery. It should be an outgrowth of a personal philosophy that balances healthy eating with healthy attitudes, healthy play with healthy habits. As we've shown, people with the best of habits are not always healthy and those with the worst habits are not always ill. Quite often the difference is attitude, passion and zest. So don't make good health serious business. Take your health seriously, but enjoy its pursuit.

12

About The Healthier Options

Our goal in writing this book has been to show people ways to build immunity. In building immunity, one minimizes the chances of succumbing to bacteria, viruses and parasites to which one is exposed. We hope we have conveyed a central point: given the role of diet, nutrition, lifestyle, hygiene, genetics, environment, attitude, stress and social factors in resistance to disease, does it make sense to merely give antibiotics when infection occurs? Hopefully this book will stimulate doctors and patients to view infection and immunity in a broader context.

In the introduction to this book, we reviewed the options one has in the care of illnesses for which antibiotics are often prescribed. The options are:

1. Use antibiotics alone. Although this is how antibiotics are usually used, it *is never* the healthier option because it does not:

- Address the underlying reasons we become sick.
- Address the side effects that can occur with antibiotic use.
- Address the bodily effect of infection itself (e.g. zinc and vitamin A loss).

Example: A child develops recurrent ear infections and is given amoxicillin only (which is typical). This is simply not enough. The doctor has not looked at the child's diet or nutritional status. Perhaps the child is allergic to cow's milk, is consuming too much sugar or is zinc deficient. The child may be on a poor diet low in

261

vitamin C and B-vitamins. Perhaps the child's ear infection followed a vaccination or viral infection, which depleted her stores of vitamin A. This would render her more susceptible to bacterial infection. Perhaps the child's parents argue incessantly, are embroiled in bitter divorce proceedings or are abusive. Less dramatically, the child may have begun day care and the separation has been stressful. Such stress commonly lowers immunity.

The above example illustrates the problem in thinking that antibiotics are the sole solution to treating infections.

2. Address the dietary, nutritional, psychological, social, lifestyle, environmental and other factors discussed in this book in conjunction with antibiotics. Used in this way, antibiotics may be the healthier option.

Example 1: A house painter suffers from recurrent sinus infections which are determined to be bacterial. He is given the antibiotic ampicillin or cefaclor. In addition, the doctor prescribes antioxidant nutrients (A, E, C, beta-carotene, selenium, etc.) that help protect the respiratory tract and sinuses from the chemicals to which the painter is exposed. The doctor also recognizes that the man has been exposed to the toxins present in paint, varnish, and solvents for years, which have made his immune system sluggish. A detoxification program is prescribed. The man is given one teaspoon of acidophilus powder three times daily to counteract the intestinal effect of the antibiotic.

Example 2: A 10-year-old boy develops a severe sore throat. The throat culture reveals that it is due to Group A beta-hemolytic streptococci. For this, an antibiotic is appropriate and is prescribed. However, the doctor also knows that the boy's nutrient stores will likely be depleted by the infection. In fact, the infection may have come about because of poor nutritional status or food intolerance. The doctor also knows that certain nutrients will help boost the activity of white blood cells needed to fight the bacteria and create a hostile environment for the bacteria. For this reason, the doctor prescribes vitamin A, E, beta-carotene, B-vitamins, selenium, echinacea and 10,000 to 20,000 milligrams of vitamin C each day. The homeopathic remedy *Belladonna* is given every two hours to relieve symptoms. The boy is given one teaspoon of acidophilus powder three times daily to counteract the intestinal effect of the antibiotic.

In both of the above examples, antibiotics were appropriate and helpful. However, the use of additional therapies would likely shorten the course of the illness, reduce complications, and improve recovery. This kind of approach takes into account many aspects of illness and treats the patient rather than the bacteria alone. This is a very important advancement in the care of infections that only a handful of doctors currently practice.

3. Address the factors discussed in this book, thereby eliminating the need for antibiotics. Sometimes, avoiding antibiotics is the healthier option.

Example 1: A 35-year-old woman develops burning when she urinates, slightly cloudy urine, and a feeling of heaviness in the bladder area. Her initial urge is to rush to the doctor for antibiotics. Yet, she knows she often develops yeast infections after such treatment. She decides to spend 24 to 48 hours treating this at home. During the initial period, she takes 2 drops of tea tree oil by mouth every 15 minutes. As symptoms improve, she extends the period of time between doses. In addition, she takes 25,000 IU of vitamin A daily and 1,000 mg of vitamin C each hour. Her symptoms begin to improve within four hours. By nightfall, she is much better. By the following evening she is nearly completely recovered.

In a case like this, many doctors and patients would have rushed to use antibiotics. However, using common sense and some simple home care remedies, the woman was able to heal under her own care.

Example 2: A 30-year-old man comes down with symptoms that include a runny nose, sneezing, watery eyes, nasal congestion, scratchy throat, headache and chills—all symptoms of the common cold. He is certain it is a cold because his wife just got over one. He avoids taking antibiotics because he knows the common cold is viral and cannot be helped by antibiotics. (Recall that roughly half of the 3 million people who saw doctors for the common cold [1983] needlessly received antibiotics.)

4. Avoid becoming sick. This is perhaps the healthiest option. If one uses some basic strategies, common illnesses can be avoided. In this way, the use of antibiotics is avoided.

Example 1: Each winter, a 50-year-old business executive suffers from repeated sore throats for which antibiotics are often prescribed. He decides he is tired of this annoying problem and begins to make changes in his life. He eliminates dairy products, sugar, ice cream, filet mignon, wine and martinis from his diet, and begins to eat more vegetables and grains. He limits his TV watching and swims for 30 minutes each day at the health club. After the swim, he takes a 15 minute sauna. He takes a multivitamin supplement with some extra antioxidants and drinks several glasses of pure water daily. To start and end each day, he spends 10 minutes doing deep breathing, relaxation exercises. This change in lifestyle brings him major improvements in health and eliminates his chronic winter sore throats. In this way, he has avoided the antibiotics that he had so frequently been given.

Example 2: A child has experienced recurrent ear infections over the past three years for which antibiotics had been repeatedly prescribed. Her parents have taken her to countless doctors, none of whom seem to offer solutions other than antibiotics and surgery. After talking to numerous other parents and reading books about alternative means of caring for childhood illness, the parents decide to take their daughter off all dairy products. After several weeks she is much improved. Several months pass and it is clear the child is having fewer problems than in the past. In the ensuing months, she is more vibrant and healthy than during any of the previous three years. As long as she limits her intake of dairy products, the child is well. The family has avoided antibiotics by keeping their daughter healthy.

Should You Say "No" When the Doctor Says "Yes"?

When confronted with evidence that antibiotics are associated with problems such as those described in this book, one is tempted to say "no" when the doctor recommends these drugs. But should you say "no" when the doctor says "yes" to antibiotics? An interesting question. Most medical authorities would say publicly that you should always follow your doctor's recommendations regarding prescription drugs and take them for the prescribed length of time. Yet, if you simply accept your doctor's advice passively, you have given up your power as an important participant in the healing journey.

Rather than saying "yes" or "no" when the doctor says "yes" to antibiotics, you may wish to explore with her many of the questions raised in this book. Are you sure it is bacterial? Are you sure it is the right antibiotic? Should a culture be performed? Are there alternatives to antibiotics? What are the risks if we don't use them? What are the risks if we wait one or two or four days? Are there dietary or nutritional factors that need consideration? Should vitamins be prescribed along with the antibiotic? Should acidophilus supplements be given to minimize the intestinal effect of the antibiotic? Could it be food allergy? Have you considered or investigated the role of food allergy?

If the problem is chronic or recurrent, you are certainly justified in getting another opinion or in seriously questioning the value and safety of the antibiotics your doctor has prescribed. Be aware, that when you approach your doctor with questions such as those mentioned above, she may not respond in the kindest tone. Many doctors do not wish to be health partners (although more are becoming interested). But it is your health in question, not theirs! Get all the answers you can.

So, should you say "no" when the doctor says "yes" to antibiotics? No. Should you ask questions and try to find the most comprehensive solution to your health problem? Absolutely.

Your Health Care Team

On November 4, 1991, an article entitled "Alternative Medicine" appeared in *Time*. A survey was reported that undoubtedly sent a wave of surprise and dismay through the medical community. The authors surveyed 500 Americans and posed three questions:

1. Have you ever sought medical help from a chiropractor, acupuncturist, herbalist, homeopathic doctor or faith healer? Thirty-one percent said they had sought care from

a chiropractor. Lesser percentages were reported for other providers (6, 5, 3, and 2 percent respectively).

2. Would you ever consider seeking medical help from an alternative doctor if conventional medicine failed to help you (among those who have not previously sought help from an alternative practitioner)? Sixty-two percent of respondents said "yes."

3. Would you go back to an alternative doctor (asked of those who had sought care from an alternative practitioner)? Eighty-four percent said "yes," reflecting a high degree of satisfaction with their care.

The results of this survey seem to reflect a growing degree of dissatisfaction with medicine as it is practiced today and a growing degree of *satisfaction* with more holistic forms of healing. This is indeed a shifting paradigm.

In addition to embracing more holistic forms of healing, patients are forcing changes in the doctor-patient relationship. The concept of the health partnership is growing in importance along with the concept of the health care team.

Many patients have developed a personal team of doctors and allied health professionals with whom they work. For certain types of problems they see their medical physician. For others, they see their chiropractor. They may also see a massage therapist, nutritionist, acupuncturist or homeopath when they feel the need. Many patients have found they are more in control of their health care decisions. These patients have begun to develop a keen ability to discern which member of the health care team to summon at which time. Also emerging from the health care team concept is the notion that the patient responds more favorably when he or she shares a common philosophy with the doctor.

The Cause of Illness

For many decades, medical scientists have pretended to know and understand the origin of many of our most common afflictions. They have also believed that they possess effective means of treating these maladies. This is especially true of "infectious" illness.

Holistic doctors have a different view of the origin of illness and of the "appropriate" treatment of illness. It is more broad and inclusive and is based upon viewing the human as a whole.

Many believe, including ourselves, that the holistic model is a more accurate and comprehensive way of viewing illness. Indeed, what we have presented here suggests that we (the authors) understand the causes of illness, the mystery of immunity, and successful means of combating disease. Yet, both the allopathic model and the holistic model (as it exists today) are incomplete.

We realize that our current understanding of this wonderful entity we call the human body, is insufficient to explain health and disease. It may be that love, forgiveness, acceptance and compassion are the true means by which wholeness and healing are brought about. Work with cancer patients, alcoholics and others suggests that higher principles may be at work. Perhaps connection to a spiritual source is the key to healing. Perhaps understanding that we are connected to one another on this planet is a key to healing.

Noted physician and author of *Space, Time and Medicine* and *Recovering the Soul,* Larry Dossey, M.D., describes three eras of medicine. Era I medicine is the medicine of the past 100 years. It is based on the reductionist idea that the body is a *machine* that becomes dysfunctional as a result of disordered chemistry or microbial invasion. The principle forms of treatment involve the prescribing of drugs and treatment by surgery. In many ways, it represents a great leap forward in our understanding and treatment of human illness. But its shortcomings become more evident as our knowledge grows.

The next era of medicine described by Dossey, Era II medicine, involves the understanding that body and mind are intricately connected. Doctors and healers are beginning to look to the mind for the healing solutions of a host of bodily ills. This model is gaining momentum and respectability. It recognizes the enormous healing potential inherent in the human mind and spirit. In fact, an entire field of medicine, psychoneuroimmunology, was spawned with this realization.

But Dossey sees an emergence to still another form of medicine, Era III. Era III is based on the recognition that we are all connected to a universal mind, a collective unconscious, as Jung called it. Dossey calls it the non-local mind. The findings of quantum physics have suggested mathematically and in some cases experimentally, that this group mind, or non-local mind exists. The study of prayer and Randolph Byrd's cardiac patients (Chapter 6) further suggests that this non-local effect exists.

The implications of Era III medicine are that ultimate healing may take place on a much grander scale than previously thought. If we all share the same mind and are part of the organism we call earth, we all share in the pain of another's illness. We all share the pain of the planet. Perhaps true healing involves a transcendence beyond ourselves—a rejection of the notion that we are alone, isolated and fundamentally different from one another. It may involve an understanding that we are each integral parts of a greater whole.

Dossey is quick to point out that the evolution to each era of medicine does not reject the truly valuable accomplishments of the former era. Emergency medicine, molecular medicine, and physical forms of healing still have a role, as does mind-body healing. The three eras of medicine will exist together in time, the best being utilized of each. As Dossey writes, "So Era III medicine does not require us to eliminate the physically based methods of Era I, or the mind-body therapies of Era II; it only adds another dimension that goes beyond their limitations."

The next great evolution in healing may come with the healing of the spirit and the heart. For some 100 years, Western society has revered the intellect. We have deified physicians and scientists—in effect, worshiped scientific achievement. In this quest for knowledge, we have lost touch with a fundamental part of ourselves—the heart. In Chinese medicine, the heart is associated with spirit. They use the term *Shen* to describe this. We use the terms "aching heart" and "broken heart" to describe deep emotional pain. Science has recently shown that the heart is inextricably linked with the mind, brain and emotions. Evidence that heart disease may be linked to the person's sense of meaning in life has also emerged. So the notion of the heart as more than a pump is a historical corollary and modern fact.

In essence, true healing recognizes the total interdependence of all body systems and strives to achieve wholeness. Symptom suppression will be viewed as a thing of the past because it denies the features that give rise to illness. In the late 21st century, scholars will likely look back at today's view of disease and treatment the same way we now view bloodletting and mercury treatments used 100 years ago.

Healing is something quite profound. Our understanding of the nature of illness and the means by which healing occurs are likely to undergo a dramatic evolution. It is the unfolding of a great mystery.

References

Chapter 1: Casualties of the War on Germs

1. Bok, D. The President's Report, 1982–83. Cambridge, Massachusetts: Harvard University, 1984.

2. Anonymous. Media-Chek. New York: International Medical News Group, 1988.

3. Hoffman, RL. Seven weeks to a settled stomach. New York: Pocket Books, 1990;6.

4. Hart, K. Corporate-funded research may be hazardous to your health. Bulletin of the Atomic Scientist 1989;45:3.

5. Anonymous. Pediatric antibiotic use soars. Medical World News 1987, November 9.

6. Wolfe, SM. Antibiotics. Health Letter. Washington, DC: The Public Citizen Health Research Group, 1989;5(7):1–5.

7. Pechere, JC, et al. Infections: recognition, understanding, treatment, Philadelphia: Lea & Febiger, 1984:37.

8. Wolfe, SM. Antibiotics. Washington, DC: Health Letter. The Public Citizen Health Research Group, 1989;5(7):1–5.

9. Galland, L, Buchman, DD. Superimmunity for kids. New York: EP Dutton, 1988;201.

10. Grundfast, K, Carney, CJ. Ear infections in your child. New York: Warner Books, 1987.

11. Cantekin, EI, McGuire, TW, Griffith, TL. Antimicrobial therapy for otitis media with effusion (secretory otitis media). JAMA 1991;266(23):3309–3317.

12. Lidefelt, KJ, Bollgren, I, Nord, CE. Changes in periurethral microflora after antimicrobial drugs. Arch Dis Child 1991;66:685–685.

13. Reid, G, et al. Vaginal flora and urinary tract infections. Current Topics in Infectious Disease 1991;4:37–41.

14. Witkin, SS. Infections in Medicine. May/June 1985:129–32.

15. Thomas, WJ, McReynolds, JW. *Haemophilus influenzae* resistant to penicillin. Lancet 1971;2:13–16.

16. Anonymous. Spread of *Haemophilus influenzae* type b. Lancet 1981;1:649.

17. Holmberg, SD, Osterholm, MT, Senger, KA, Cohen, ML. Drug-resistant Salmonella from animals fed antimicrobials. N Engl J Med 1984;311(10).

18. Pechere, JC, et al.:44.

19. Jaffe, R. Personal communication, 1991.

20. McKeown, T. The role of medicine: dream, mirage or nemesis. Princeton, NJ: Princeton University Press, 1979;107.

Chapter 2: Antibiotics:
What Your Doctor May Not Tell You

1. McKeown, T. The role of medicine: dream, mirage or nemesis. Oxford University Press, 1976;391.

2. Dixon, B. Beyond the magic bullet: the real story of medicine. New York: Harper & Row, 1978;64

3. Hume, ED. Pasteur exposed: the false foundations of modern medicine. Australia: Bookreal, 1989.

4. Lappé, M. When antibiotics fail: restoring the ecology of the body. Berkeley, CA: North Atlantic Books, 1986:17–18.

5. McKeown, T.:391

6. McKeown, T.:62.

7. Kass, EH. Infectious diseases and social change. J Infect Dis 1971;123(1):110–114.

8. McKinlay, JB, McKinlay, SM. The questionable contribution of medical measures to the decline of mortality in the United States in the twentieth century. *Millbank Memorial Fund Quarterly* Summer 1977;405–428.

9. McKinlay, JB, McKinlay, SM.:422.

References

10. McKinlay, JB, McKinlay, SM.:423.

11. Lappé, M.:18.

12. Weinstein, L. Infectious disease: retrospect and reminiscence. J Infect Dis 1974; 129(4):480–92.

13. Anonymous. Those overworked miracle drugs. Newsweek 1981;8(17):63.

14. Schmidt, MA. Childhood ear infections: what every parent and physician should know. Berkeley, CA: North Atlantic Books, 1990.

15. Welch, GH. Antibiotic resistance: a new kind of epidemic. Postgraduate Medicine 1984;76(6).

16. Drug Information. American Hospital Formulary Service, Bethesda, Maryland: American Society of Hospital Pharmacists, Inc., 1986;218.

17. Thomas, WJ, McReynolds, JW. *Haemophilus influenzae* resistant to penicillin. Lancet 1971;2:13–16.

18. Schwartz, R, Rodriguez, W, Khan, W, Ross, S. The increasing incidence of ampicillin-resistant *Haemophilus influenzae:* a cause of otitis media. JAMA 1978;239(4).

19. Schwarcz, SK, et al. National surveillance of antimicrobial resistance in *Neisseria gonorrhoeae.* JAMA 1990;264:1413–1417.

20. Crook, WG. The yeast connection. New York: Vintage Books, 1986;133.

21. Cohen, SR, Thompson, JW. Otitic candidiasis in children: an evaluation of the problem and effectiveness of ketoconazole in 10 patients. Ann Otol Rhinol Laryngol 1990;99:427–31.

22. Witkin, SS. Infections in Medicine. May/June 1985:129–32.

23. Crook, WG. Chronic fatigue syndrome and the yeast connection. Jackson, TN: Professional Books, Inc. 1992;319.

24. Crook, WG.:340.

25. Bauman, DS, Hagglund, HE. Polysystem chronic complainers. J Adv Med 1991;4(1).

26. Hauser, WE, Remington, JS. Effect of antibiotics on the

immune response. Am J Med 1982;72(5):711–15.

27. Pichichero, M, Disney, FA, Talpey, WB, et al. Adverse and beneficial effects of immediate treatment of group A beta hemolytic streptococcal pharyngitis with penicillin. Ped Infect Dis J 1987;6:635–643.

28. Diamant, M, Diamant, B. Abuse and timing of antibiotics in acute otitis media. Arch Otolaryngol 1974;100:226–232.

29. Cantekin, EI, McGuire, TW, Griffith, TL. Antimicrobial therapy for otitis media with effusion (secretory otitis media). JAMA 1991;266(23):3309–3317.

30. Lappé, M.:54.

31. Galland, L. Nurrition and candidiasis. J Orthomolecular Psych 1985;14(1):50–60.

32. Archer, M. J Env Hlth 1989.

33. Ward, NI, et al. The influence of the chemical additive tartrazine on the zinc status of hyperactive children- a double-blind placebo-controlled study. J Nutr Med 1990;1:51–7.

34. Kumar, A, Weatherly, MR, Beaman, DC. Sweeteners, flavorings and dyes in antibiotic preparations. Pediatrics 1991;87(3).

35. Klein, JO. Microbiology of otitis media. Ann Otol Rhinol Laryngol 1980;89(Suppl 68):98.

36. Chaput de Saintonge, DM, Levine, DF. Trial of three-day and ten-day courses of amoxycillin in otitis media. Br Med J 1982;284:1078–1081.

37. Bain, J, Murphy, E, Ross, F. Acute otitis media: clinical course among children who received a short course of high dose antibiotic. Br Med J 1985;291:1243–1246.

38. Hendrickse, WA, Kusmiesz, H, et al. Five vs. ten days of therapy for acute otitis media. Pediatr Inf Dis J 1988;7:14–23.

39. Meistrup-Larsen, KI, Sorenson, H, et al. Two versus seven days penicillin treatment for acute otitis media. Acta Otolaryngol 1983;96:99–104.

References

40. Hendrickse, WA, et al:14–23.

41. Meistrup-Larsen, KI, et al:99–104.

42. The physician's desk reference. Oradell, NJ: Medical Economics Company, 1990.

43. Anonymous. Pediatric antibiotic use soars. Medical World News 1987, November 9.

44. Skoner, DP, Stillwagon, PK, et al. Inflammatory mediators in chronic otitis media with effusion. Arch Otolaryngol Head Neck Surg 1988;114:1131–33.

45. Neu, HC, Howrey, SP. Testing the physician's knowledge of antibiotic use. N Engl J Med 1975;293:1291.

46. The physician's desk reference.

47. Hart, K. Corporate-funded research may be hazardous to your health. Bulletin of the Atomic Scientist 45;3:1989.

48. Anonymous, Policing the page [Editorial]. Economist 1989, June 3:119.

49. Cantekin, EI, McGuire, TW, Griffith, TL. Antimicrobial therapy for otitis media with effusion (secretory otitis media). JAMA 1991;266(23):3309–3317.

50. US Special Committee on Aging: Aging America. Trends and projections. 1987–88 edition. U.S. Department of Health and Human Services No. LR 3377(188)-D12198.

51. Kasper, JA. Prescribed medicines; Uses, expenditures, and source of payment (Preview 9, National Health Care Expenditure Study) Washington, D.C., U.S. Department of Health and Human Services, DHHS publication No. (PHS) 82–3320, 1982.

52. Cummings, DM, Uttech, KM. Antibiotics for common infections in the elderly. Primary care: infectious diseases 1990;17(4):887.

53. Lancet, September 27, 1986.

54. Penn, ND, Purkins, L, Kelleher, J, Heatley, RV, Mascie-Taylor, BH, Belfield, PW. The effect of dietary supplementation with vitamins A, C and E on cell-mediated immune function in elderly long-stay patients: a randomized

controlled trial. Age and Ageing 1991;20:169–174.

55. Anonymous. Pediatric antibiotic use soars. Medical World News 1987, November 9:8.

56. Hagerman, RJ, Falkenstein, AR. An association between recurrent otitis media in infancy and later hyperactivity. Clin Ped 1987;26(5).

57. Lidefelt, KJ, et al. Changes in periurethral microflora after antimicrobial drugs. Archives of Diseases in Childhood, 66;1991:683–685.

58. Crook, WG. The yeast connection. New York: Vintage Books, 1986;214.

59. Crook, WG.:214–15.

60. Castle, M, Wilfet, CM, Cate, TR, Osterhout, S. Antibiotic use at Duke University Medical Center. JAMA 1977, June 27.

61. Anonymous. Most antibiotic misuse linked to use as prophylaxis in surgery. Internal Medicine News 1983;1:1.

62. Wang, J. Antibiotic prophylaxis in surgery: too much or not enough? Modern Medicine 1975;43(15):40.

63. Kheel, M. Townsend Letter for Doctors 1992;2.

64. Beasley, JD, Swift, JJ. The Kellog Report. Annandale-on-Hudson, NY: The Institute of Health Policy and Practice, 1989;305.

65. American Heart Association. Preventing bacterial endocarditis: a statement for the dental profession. JAMA 1990;264(22):2919–22.

66. van der Meer, JTM, et al. Efficacy of antibiotic prophylaxis for prevention of native-valve endocarditis. Lancet 1992;339:135–139.

67. Wall Street Journal 1989, October 2.

68. Neu, HC, Howrey, SP. Testing the physician's knowledge of antibiotic use. N Engl J Med 1975;293:1291.

69. Chandler, D, Dugdale, AE. What do patients know about antibiotics? Br Med J 1976;8:422.

References

70. Inlander, CB, Levin, LS, Weiner, E. Medicine on trial: the appalling story of medical ineptitude and the arrogance that overlooks it. New York: Pantheon Books, 1988;70 (This study is reviewed.)

71. Poses, RM, Cebul, RD, et al. The accuracy of experienced physicians' probability estimates for patients with sore throats. JAMA 1985;254(7):927.

72. Wang, T, Tiessen, E. Canadian Family Physician 1989 35:1771.

73. Pechere, JC, et al. Infection: recognition, understanding, treatment. Philadelphia: Lea & Febiger, 1984:37.

74. Jaffe, DM. High fever: is early antibiotic treatment useful? N Engl J Med 1987;317:1175.

75. Bakwin, R., quoted in Scheff, TJ. Decision rules and their consequences. Behaviour Science 1963;97–107.

76. Disney, FA. Pediatricians, antibiotics, and office practice. Pediatrics 1984;75:1135.

77. Neu, HC, Howrey, SP. Testing the physician's knowledge of antibiotic use. N Engl J Med 1975;293:1291.

78. Hughes, R, Brewin, R. The tranquilizing of America. New York: Harcourt Brace Jovanovich, 1979.

79. Melville, A, Johnson, C. Cured to death: the effects of prescription drugs. New York: Stein and Day, 1982;176 (Hughes is reviewed.)

80. Marks, JH, Goldberg, DP, Hillier, VF. Determinants of the ability of general practitioners to detect psychiatric illness. Psychological Medicine 1979; 9:337–53.

81. Melville, A, Johnson, C. Cured to death: the effects of prescription drugs. New York: Stein and Day, 1982;183.

82. Berkow, S, Palmer, S. Nutrition in medical education: current status and future directions. Food and Nutrition Board, National Research Council, National Academy of Sciences, 2101 Constitution Avenue N.W., Washington, D.C., 20418.

83. Crook, WG, Stevens, L. Solving the puzzle of your hard to raise child. New York: Random House, 1987;132.

84. Crook, WG.:153.

85. Gaby, A. Vitamin C potentiates antibiotic therapy. Townsend Letter for Doctors 1990;523.

Chapter 3: The Miracle of Immunity

1. Behar, M. A deadly combination. *World Health* Feb-Mar, 1974;29.

2. Jaret, P. Our immune system: the wars within. *National Geographic* 1986;169(6):702–733.

3. Levine, S. Healing into life and death. New York: Anchor Books, 1987;197.

4. Soll, D. University of Iowa, Personal communication, 1990.

Chapter 4: Food, Nutrition and Infection Susceptibility

1. Newberne, PM, Williams, G. Nutritional influences on the course of infections. In Dunlop, RH, Moon, HW. Resistance to infectious disease. Saskatoon, Canada: Saskatoon Modern Press, 1970;93.

2. Kalokorinos, A, Dettman, G. A supportive submission, In The dangers of immunization, Biological Research Institute, Warburton, Victoria, Australia 1979;68. (Originally written and published by the Humanitarian Society in Quakertown, PA, and enlarged and republished by the Biological Research Institute, Australia.)

3. Dixon, B. Beyond the magic bullet: the real story of medicine. New York: Harper & Row, 1978;64.

4. Newberne, PM, Williams, G. Nutritional influences on the course of infections. In Dunlop, RH, Moon, HW. Resistance to infectious disease. Saskatoon, Canada: Saskatoon Modern Press, 1970;93.

5. McKeown, T. The role of medicine: dream, mirage or nemesis. Princeton, NJ: Princeton University Press, 1979:75.

6. McKeown, T.:60.

7. Chavance, M, et al. Nutritional support improves antibody response to influenza virus in the elderly. Br Med J

References

1985;11(9):1348–49.

8. Nockels, CF. Protective effects of supplemental vitamin E against infection. Fed Proc 1979;38:2134–8.

9. Willmott, F, et al. Lancet 1983;1:1053.

10. Freinberg, N, Lyte, T. Adjunctive ascorbic acid administration and antibiotic therapy. J Dent Res 1957;36:260–62.

11. Schachner, L, et al. A clinical trial comparing the safety and efficacy of topical erythromycin-zinc formulation with a topical Clindamycin formulation. J Am Acad Dermatol 1990;22(3)489–95.

12. Campos, FA, Flores, H, Underwood, BA. Effect of an infection on vitamin A status of children as measured by the relative dose response (RDR). Am J Clin Nutr 1987;46:91–4.

13. Frieden, TR, Sowell, AL, Henning, KJ, Huff, DL, Gunn, RA. Vitamin A levels and severity of measles. Am J Dis Child 1992;146:182–86.

14. Horrobin, DF. Essential fatty acids and the post-viral fatigue syndrome. In Jenkins, R, Mowbray, J. (eds), Post-viral fatigue syndrome. New York: John Wiley & Sons, 1991;393–404.

15. Breneman, JC. Basics of food allergy. Springfield, Illinois: Charles C. Thomas, 1978:8.

16. Anonymous. Says food allergy seems important cause of otitis. Family Pract News 1991;21(5):14.

17. Crook, WG. Food allergy- the great masquerader. Ped Clin North Am 1975;22(1):227–38.

18. Naunton, E. Miami Herald, 1988, Nov. 12.

19. Rowe, AH. Clinical allergy. Philadelphia: Lea & Febiger, 1937.

20. Dostaolova, L. Dev Pharmacol Ther 1982;4(Suppl. 1):45.

21. Bogden, JD, et al. Zinc and immunocompetence in the elderly: baseline data on zinc nutriture and immunity in unsupplemented subjects. Am J Clin Nutr 1987;46(1): 101–09.

22. Sanstead, HH. Am J Clin Nutr 1973;26:1251–60.

23. Werbach, MR. Nutritional influences on mental illness. Tarzana, CA: Third Line Press, Inc., 1991:267.

24. Galland, L, Buchnan, D. SuperImmunity for kids. New York: E.P. Dutton, 1988:12.

25. Werbach, MR.:255–71.

26. Beasley, J, Swift, J. The Kellogg report: The impact of environment & lifestyle on the health of Americans. Annandale-on-Hudson, NY: The Bard College Center, 1989;144.

27. DeSchepper, L. Peak Immunity. Santa Monica, CA: Self-published. 1989;25.

28. Newberne, PM. Over-nutrition on resistance of dogs to distemper virus. Fedn Proc 1966;25:1701–1710.

29. Sandler, BP. Diet prevents polio, The Lee Foundation for Nutritional Research, 1951;43.

30. Sanchez, A, et al. Role of sugars in human neutrophilic phagocytosis. Am J Clin Nutr 1973;26:180.

31. Stitt, PA. Fighting the food giants. Manitowoc, Wisconsin: Natural Press, 1980.

32. Stitt, PA.:144.

33. Select Committee On Nutrition and Human Needs, United States Senate. Dietary Goals for the United States. Washington: United States Government Printing Office, 1977.

34. US News and World Report 1985;July 15.

35. Northwest Airlines World Traveler, Compass Readings. 1991;2:46.

36. Philpott, WH, Kalita, DK. Brain allergies: the psychonutrient connection. New Canaan, Connecticut: Keats Publishing, Inc., 1980;20.

37. Hoffman, RL. Seven weeks to a settled stomach. New York: Pocket Books, 1990;6.

38. Dagnelie, P, van Staveren, W, van den Berg, H. Vitamin B_{12}

from algae appears not to be bioavailable. Am J Clin Nutr 1991;53:695–7.

39. Hussey, GD, Kelin, M. A randomized, controlled trial of vitamin A in children with severe measles. N Engl J Med 1990;323:160–4.

40. Bauernfeind, JC. The safe use of vitamin A: a report of the International Vitamin A Consultative Group. Washington, D.C.: The Nutrition Foundation, 1980.

41. Anderson, R. Ascorbate-mediated stimulation of neutrophil motility and lymphocyte transformation by inhibition of the peroxidase-H_2O_2–halide system in vitro and in vivo. Am. J Clin Nutr. 1981; 34:1906–11.

42. Chandra, RK. Excessive zinc impairs immune responses. JAMA 1984;252(11):1443–46.

43. Anneren, G, Magnusson, CGM, Nordvall, SL. Increase in serum concentrations of IgG2 and IgG4 by selenium supplementation in children with Down's Syndrome. Arch Dis Child. 1990;65:1353–55.

44. Bliznakov, EG, Hunt, GL. The miracle nutrient: coenzyme Q_{10}. New York: Bantam Books, 1987;64.

Chapter 5:
Environmental Threats to a Healthy Immune System

1. Speirs, RS, Roberts, DW, Hinsdill, RD, Speirs, EE. A holistic approach to in vivo immunotoxicity testing. FDA 1980;55–59.

2. Hunnisett, A, Howard, J, Davies, S. Gut fermentation (or the "auto-brewery") syndrome: a new clinical test with initial observations and discussion of clinical and biochemical implications. J Nutr Med 1990;1:33–38.

3. Huggins, HA, Huggins, SA. It's all in your head. Colorado Springs: Self-published, 1985;41.

4. Summers, AO, Wireman, J, Totis, PA, Blankenship, J, Vimy, MF, Lorscheider, FL. Mercury released from dental "silver" fillings increases the incidence of multiply resistant bacteria in the oral and intestinal normal flora. American Society for

References

Microbiology Annual Meeting, Dallas, TX 1991;A-137.

5. Christiansen, G. Clinical Research Associates Newsletter 1990;14(12).

6. Becker, RO, Selden, G. The body electric: electromagnetism and the foundation of life. New York: William Morrow Company, Inc., 1985:293.

7. Becker, RO.:293.

8. Rogers, SA. The EI Syndrome: An Rx for Environmental Illness. Syracuse, NY: Prestige Publishers, 1986:171.

9. Chilmonczyk, B. Environmental tobacco smoke exposure during infancy. Am J Pub Hlth 1990;80(10):1205–08.

10. Laseter, JL, DeLeon, IR, Rea, WJ, Butler, JR. Chlorinated hydrocarbon pesticides in environmentally sensitive patients. Clinical Ecology 1983;2(1):10.

11. Mendell, MJ, Smith, AH. Consistent pattern of elevated symptoms in air-conditioned office buildings: a reanalysis of epidemiologic studies. Am J Pub Hlth, 1990;80:1193–1199.

12. Dales, RE, et al. Respiratory health effects of home dampness and molds among Canadian children. Am J Pub Hlth 1991;134(2):196–203.

13. Dixon, B. Beyond the magic bullet: the real story of medicine. New York: Harper & Row, 1978;137.

14. Beasley, J, Swift, J. The Kellogg report: The impact of environment & lifestyle on the health of Americans. Annandale-on-Hudson, NY: The Bard College Center, 1989;243.

15. Allen, FE. One man's suffering spurs doctors to probe pesticide-drug link. Wall St J 1991;Oct 14:A1.

16. Bland, JS. Pesticide-drug link. Preventive Medicine Update 1992;12(1).

17. Tretjak, Z, Shields, M, Beckman, S. PCB reduction and clinical improvement by detoxification: an unexploited approach. Human & Experimental Toxicology 1990;9:235–44.

18. Bland, JS. Personal communication, 1991.

19. Conference Proceedings. Nutrition as it relates to environmental medicine. American Academy of Environmental Medicine, Minneapolis, Minnesota, July 25, 26, 1990:150.

Chapter 6: Heredity and Lifestyle

1. Beasley, J, Swift, J. The Kellogg report: The impact of environment & lifestyle on the health of Americans. Annandale-on-Hudson, NY: The Bard College Center, 1989;243.

2. DeCosse, JJ, Miller, HH, Lesser, ML. Effect of wheat fiber and vitamins C and E on rectal polyps in patients with familial adenomatous polyposis. J Natl Cancer Inst 1989;81:1290–7.

3. Anneren, G, Magnusson, CGM, Nordvall, SL. Increase in serum concentrations of IgG2 and IgG4 by selenium supplementation in children with Down's Syndrome. Arch Dis Child 1990;65:1353–55.

4. Boxer, LA, Watanabe, AM, et al. Correction of leukocyte function in Chediak-Higashi Syndrome by ascorbate. N Engl J Med 1976;295:1041–45.

5. Dixon, B. Beyond the magic bullet. New York: Harper & Row, 1978;67.

6. Williams, RJ, Deason, G. Individuality in vitamin C needs. Proc Nat Acad Sci 1968; 57:1638.

7. Williams, RJ, Pelton, RB. Individuality in nutrition: effects of vitamin A-deficient and other deficient diets on experimental animals. Proc Nat Acad Sci 1966;55:126.

8. Williams, RJ. Nutrition against disease. New York: Pitman Publishing Corporation, 1971:24.

9. Geschwind, N, Galaburda, A. Biological foundations of cerebral dominance Cambridge: Harvard University Press, 1984.

10. Beach, R, Gershwin, M, Hurley, L. Persistent immunological consequences of gestational zinc deprivation. Am J Clin Nutr 1982;35 (Suppl):579–90.

References

11. Ames, B. Proc Nat Acad Sci 1991;11003.

12. Dostaolova, L. *Dev Pharmacol Ther* 1982;4(Suppl. 1):45.

13. McKeown, T. The role of medicine: dream, mirage or nemesis? Princeton, NJ: Princeton University Press, 1979;180.

14. Weatherford, J. Indian givers: how the Indians of the Americas transformed the world. New York: Fawcett Columbine, 1988;189–90.

15. Kauppinen, K, Vuori, I. Man in the sauna. Ann Clin Res 1986;18:173–85.

16. Hollwich, F, Dieckhues, B. The effect of natural and artificial light via the eye on the hormonal and metabolic balance of animal and man. Opthalmologica 1980;180(4):188–197.

17. Belyayev, II, et al. Combined use of ultraviolet radiation to control acute respiratory disease. Vestn Akad Med Nauk 1975;SSSR3:37.

18. Dantsig, NM. Ultraviolet radiation. In Russian language book. Moscow: 1966.

19. Zabaluyeva, AP. General immunological reactivity of the organism in prophylactic ultraviolet irradiation of children in northern regions. Vestn Akad Med Nauk 1975;3:23.

20. Harmon, DB. The coordinated classroom. Grand Rapids, Michigan: American Seating Company, 1951.

21. Castleman, M. Cold cures. New York: Fawcett Columbine, 1987:57–8.

22. Journal of Dentistry for Children 1989;56(3):201–204.

23. Schectman, G, Byrd, J, Hoffmann, R. Ascorbic acid requirements for smokers: analysis of a population survey. Am J Clin Nutr 1991;53:1466–70.

24. Tucker, LA, Bagwell, M. Television viewing and obesity in adult females. Am J Pub Hlth 1991;81(7):908–911.

25. Nieman, DC, Nehlsen-Cannarella, SL, Markoff, PA, et al. The effects of moderate exercise training on natural killer-cells and acute upper respiratory tract infections. Int J Sports Med 1990;11(6):467–73.

References

26. Hippocrates News 1991;10(2).

27. Peters, EM, Bateman, ED. Ultramarathon running and upper respiratory tract infections: an epidemiology survey. SA Med J 1983;64:582–584.

28. Smith, L. Personal communication. Unpublished research, 1991.

29. Beecher, MM. Three cardiologists report prayers for their patients are answered. Medical Tribune 1986; Jan. 8:3–15,.

30. Owen, R. Qualitative research: the early years. Salem, Oregon: Grayhaven Books, 1988:22–3.

31. Hamburg, DA, Elliott, GR, Parron, DL. Health and behavior: frontiers of research in the biobehavioral sciences. Washington, DC: National Academy Press, 1982.

32. Dixon, B. Beyond the magic bullet. New York: Harper & Row, 1978;65. (Paget is quoted.)

33. Krueger, JM, Karnovsky, ML. Sleep and the immune response. Annals of the New York Academy of Science 1987;496:510–16.

34. Hauri, P. The sleep disorders. In Current Concepts. The Upjohn Company, 1982.

35. New Age Journal 1990;Nov/Dec:9–10.

36. Montague, A. Touching: the human significance of the skin. New York: Harper & Row, 1978;188.

37. Montague, A.:188.

38. Tisserand, R. Aromatherapy: to heal and tend the body. Santa Fe, New Mexico: Lotus Press, 1988:56–57.

39. Cohen, S. Sound effects on behavior. Psychology Today 1981;10:38–49.

40. Bottom Line and Personal, 1991;12(8):15.

41. Kiecolt-Glaser, JK, Glaser, R, et al. Modulation of cellular immunity in medical students. J Behavior Med 1986;9(1):5–21.

42. van Breda, W, van Breda, J. A comparative study of the health status of children raised under the health care models

of chiropractic and allopathic medicine. J Chir Res
1989(Summer):101–3.

43. Sobel, D, Ornstein, R. Healthy pleasures. Reading,
Massachusetts: Addison Wesley, 1989.

Chapter 7: Mood, Mind, Stress and Infections

1. Justice, B. Who gets sick. Los Angeles: Jeremy P. Tarcher,
Inc., 1988:171.

2. Sachs, BC. Coping with stress. Stress Medicine 1991;7:61–63.

3. Locke, S, Colligan, D. The healer within. New York: New
American Library, 1986;71.

4. Ferguson, M, Coleman, W, Perrin, P. PragMagic. New York:
Pocket Books, 1990;151.

5. Sehnert, KW. Stress/unstress. Minneapolis: Augsburg
Publishing House, 1981;19.

6. Locke, S, Colligan, D. The healer within. New York: New
American Library, 1986;68.

7. Boyce, TW, et al. Influence of life events and family routines
on childhood respiratory tract illness. Pediatrics
1977;60(4):609–615.

8. Meyer, RJ, Haggerty, RJ. Streptococcal infections in families.
Pediatrics 1962;4:539–49.

9. Selye, H. The stress of life. New York: McGraw Hill,
1978:299.

10. Cassata, DM. Personal communication. Bloomington,
Minnesota, 1990.

11. Cohen, S, Tyrrell, D, Smith, A. Psychological stress and
susceptibility to the common cold. New Engl J Med
1991;325:606–12.

12. Cohen, S, et al.:606.

13. Dossey, L. Black Monday. New Age 1991;Nov/Dec:36,
100–101.

14. Dossey, L.:100–101.

15. Ferguson, M, Coleman, W, Perrin, P. PragMagic. New York:

References

Pocket Books, 1990;106.

16. Pennebaker, JW, Burnam, MA, Schaeffer, MA, Harper, DC. Lack of control as a determinant of perceived physical symptoms. J Personal Soc Psych 1977;35(3):167–74.

17. Slovut, G. Great expectations: elderly who call selves healthy may live longer. Star Tribune 1991;April 16.

18. Idler, E, Kasl, S. Journal of Gerontology: Social Sciences March 1991.

19. Justice, B. Who gets sick: how thoughts, moods and beliefs can affect your health. Los Angeles: J.P. Tarcher, 1988.

20. Peterson, C. Explanatory style as a risk factor for illness. Cognitive Therapy Research 1988;12:117–30. See also Peterson, C. Journal of Personality and Social Psychology.

21. Sobel, D, Ornstein, R. Healthy pleasures. Reading, Massachusetts: Addison Wesley, 1989;168.

22. Seligman, MEP. Learned optimism. New York: Alfred A. Knopf, 1991;167–184.

23. Locke, S, Colligan, D. The healer within. New York: New American Library, 1986;68.

224. Kasl, SV, Evans, AS, Neiderman, JC. Psychosocial risk factors in the development of infectious mononucleosis. Psychosomatic Medicine 1979;41:445–66.

25. Women abused as kids found in poorer health. The New York Times, August 1990.

26. Bandura, A. Self-efficacy mechanism in human agency. American Psychologist 1982;37:122–47.

27. Moskowitz, H. Hiding in the Hammond Report. Hospital Practice 1975;8:35–39.

28. Marmot, M, Syme, SL. Acculturation and coronary heart disease in Japanese-Americans. American Journal of Epidemiology 1976;104:107–23.

29. Sobel, D, Ornstein, R. Healthy pleasures. Reading, Massachusetts: Addison Wesley, 1989.

30. Angier, N. Chronic anger is major health risk: studies find.

References

The New York Times, 1990;Dec. 13. Papers presented at a
1990 conference of the American Heart Association.

31. Angier, N.

32. Williams, R. The Trusting Heart: Great News About Type A
    Behavior. New York: Times Books, 1989. (Quoted in
    Pragmagic, Ferguson, M., et al. New York: Pocket Books,
    1990;150.)

33. Thomsen, J, Bretlau, P, et al. Placebo effect for surgery for
    Meniere's disease. Arch Otolaryngol 1981;107;271–77.

34. Thomsen, Bretlau, et al. Placebo effect in surgery for
    Meniere's disease: three-year follow-up. Otolaryngology
    Head Neck Surgery 1983;91:183.

35. Wolf, S. The pharmacology of placebos. Pharmacological
    Reviews 1959;11:689–704.

36. Adler, G. The physician and the hypochondrial patient. New
    Engl J Med 1981;June 4:1394–96.

37. Giving Mirth. Mothering 1990;Winter.

38. Cousins, N. Anatomy of an illness. New York: WW Norton,
    1979.

39. The American Heritage Dictionary of the English Language.
    Boston: Houghton Mifflin Company, 1976.

40. Mind-Body-Health Digest 1990;2:5.

41. Dillon, KM, Minchoff, B, Baker, KH. Positive emotional
    states and enhancement of the immune system. International
    Journal of Psychiatry in Medicine 1985–86;15:13–17.

42. Chopra, D. Quantum Healing. New York: Bantam Books,
    1989;67.

43. Dreher, H. Are you immune-competent? East West Natural
    Health 1992;1:52–59.

44. Bagne, P. Dark heart. Omni 1988;Oct:34, 214.

45. Williams, R. The trusting heart. New Age Journal 1989;May-
    June:26–30.

Chapter 8:
Vitamin C: Powerful Preventive and Treatment

1. Pauling, L. How to live longer and feel better. New York: W.H. Freeman, 1986:127.

2. Pauling, L. Vitamin C and the common cold. San Francisco: W.F. Freeman and Co., 1970.

3. Carpenter, KJ. The history of scurvy and vitamin C. New York: Cambridge University Press, 1986.

4. Bessley, J, Swift, J. The Kellogg report: the impact of environment & lifestyle on the health of Americans. Annandale-on-Hudson, NY: The Bard College Center, 1989.

5. Schectman, G, et al. Ascorbic acid requirement for smokers: analysis of a population survey. Am J Clin Nutr 1991;53:1466–70.

6. Klein, MA. The National Cancer Institute and ascorbic acid. Townsend Letter for Doctors 1991;12:967–70.

7. Beasley, J, et al. 1989.

8. Klenner, FR. Virus pneumonia and its treatment with vitamin C. So Med Surg 1948;2.

9. Klenner, FR. Massive doses of vitamin C and the virus diseases. J So Med Surg 1951;113(4).

10. Klenner, FR. Observations on the dose and administration of ascorbic acid when employed beyond the range of a vitamin in human pathology. J Appl Nutr 1971;23:3–4.

11. Klenner, FR. The use of vitamin C as an antibiotic. J Appl Nutr 1953;6.

12. Kalokerinos, A. Every Second Child. New Canaan, Connecticut: Keats Publishing, 1981.

13. deWit, JC. JAMA 1950;144:879.

14. Stone, I. The healing factor: vitamin C against disease. New York: Grosset and Dunlap, 1972.

15. Pauling, L. How to live longer and feel better. New York: W.H. Freeman, 1986.

References

16. McCall, CE, Cooper, R. Vitamin C shows promise as a bactericidal agent. Bowman Gray School Med, Med Alumni News 1972;14:1.

17. Pauling, L. How to live longer and feel better. New York: W.H. Freeman, 1986.

18. Hume, P, Wyers, E. Changes in leukocyte ascorbic acid during the common cold. Scottish Med J 1973;18:3–7.

19. Asfora, J. Vitamin C in high doses in the treatment of the common cold. In Hanck, A, Ritzel, G. (eds.). Re-evaluation of vitamin C. Bern: Hans Huber, 1977:219–34.

20. Prinz, W, Bortz, R, Bragin, B, Hersch, M. The effect of ascorbic acid supplementation on some parameters of the human immunological defence system. Intl J Vit Nutr Res 1977;47:248–56.

21. Klein, MA. The National Cancer Institute and ascorbic acid. Townsend Letter for Doctors 1991;12:967–70.

22. Klenner, FR. Massive doses of vitamin C and the virus diseases. J So Med Surg 1951;113(4).

23. Klenner, FR. Massive doses.

24. Klenner, FR. Massive doses.

25. Cheraskin, E. Health and happiness. Wichita, Kansas: Biocommunications Press, 1989;70.

26. Jungeblut, CW. Vitamin C therapy and prophylaxis in experimental poliomyelitis. J Exper Med 1937;65:127.

27. Rivers, JM. Safety of high-level vitamin C ingestion. Applied nutrition, Third conference on vitamin C, Ann NY Acad Sci 1987;498:445–454.

28. Hornig, D. Safety of vitamin and mineral supplements for mother and child. In Berger, H. (ed). Vitamins and minerals in pregnancy and lactation. Nestle' nutrition workshop series. New York: Raven Press, Ltd., 1988;16:433–4.

29. Cheraskin, E, Ringsdorf, WM. The vitamin C connection. New York: Harper and Row, 1983;201–19.

30. Klein, MA. The National Cancer Institute and ascorbic acid. Townsend Letter for Doctors 1991;12:967–70.

31. Klein, MA.:967–70.

Chapter 9: Boosting Immunity Naturally: Complementary Treatments Old and New

1. Glasser, RJ. The Body is the Hero. New York: Random House, 1976.

2. Hodgin, D. Seeking Cures in the Jungle. Insight 1991;10:30–1.

3. Mowrey, DB. The scientific validation of herbal medicine. Cormorant Books, 1986:250.

4. Foster, S. Echinacea: nature's immune enhancer. Rochester, Vermont: Healing Arts Press, 1991:39–60.

5. Mowrey, DB.:122.

6. Hunan Medical College, China. Garlic in cryptococcal meningitis: a preliminary report of 21 cases. Chinese Medical Journal 1980;93:123–6.

7. Fortunatov, MN. Experimental use of phytoncides for therapeutic and prophylactic purposes. Voprosy Pediatril i Okhrany Materinstva: Detstva 1952;20(2):55–8.

8. Cavallito, CJ, Bailey, JH. Allicin, the antibacterial principle of allium sativum: isolation, physical properties and antibacterial action. J Am Oil Chem Soc 1945;66:1950–51.

9. Mowrey, DB.:158.

10. Mano, D. Studies on the inhibitory action of plant (licorice root) components on the growth of bacteria: a study on the inhibitory action of radix liquiritiae fractions on bacterial growth and the increased potential of resistance in bacteria. Japanese J Bact 1962;17(12):938–41.

11. Aoki, T, et al. Low natural killer cell syndrome: clinical and immunological features. Nat Immun Cell Growth Regul 1987;6:116–28.

12. Schnaubelt, K. Aromatherapy Course. San Rafael, CA: Pacific Institute of Aromatherapy, 1987;16–18.

13. Schnaubelt, K.:9.

14. Schnaubelt, K.:8.

References

15. Rideal, EK, et al. Perfume Record 1930;21:344. (Cited in, Gildemeister, E, Hoffmann, FR. The essential oils, (Treibs, W. [ed]) Berlin: Akademie Verlag, 4th edition 1956;1:129.)

16. Schnaubelt, K.:8.

17. Rommelt, H, et al. Zeitschrift f. Phytotherapie 1988;9:11–13.

18. Kar, A, Jain, SR. Antibacterial evaluation of some indigenous medicinal volatile oils. Qual Plant Mater Veg 1971;20(3):231–7.

19. Gattefossé, HM. article in Perfumery and Essential Oil Record 1954;12:406–9.

20. Liu, SL. Therapeutic effects of borneol-walnut oil in the treatment of purulent otitis media. Chinese Journal of Integrated Traditional and Western Medicine (Beijing) 1990;10(2):93–5.

21. Kaptchuk, T, Croucher, M. The healing arts. London, 1986.

22. Tisserand, RB. The art of aromatherapy. Rochester, Vermont: Healing Arts Press, 1977.

23. Tisserand, RB.:320.

24. Bradford, T. The logic of figures or comparative results of homeopathic and other treatments. Philadelphia: Boericke & Tafel, 1900.

25. Ullman, D. Homeopathy: medicine for the twenty-first century. Berkeley, California: North Atlantic Books, 1988;126–7.

26. Bradford, T. 1900.

27. Coulter, H. Divided legacy: the conflict between homeopathy and the American Medical Association. Berkeley, California: North Atlantic Books, 1973;3:302.

28. Ullman, D.:126–7.

29. Castro, D, Nogueira, GG. Use of the nosode Menigococcinum as a preventive against meningitis. J Am Inst Homeop 1975;68:211–219.

30. Gaucher, C, Jeulin, D, Peycru, P. Homeopathic treatment of cholera in Peru: an initial clinical study. Brit Homeop J 1992;81:18–21.

31. Brennan, PC, Hondras, MA. Priming of neutrophils for enhanced respiratory burst by manipulation of the thoracic spine. Proceedings of the International Conference on Spinal Manipulation 1989;160–3.

32. Gutmann, G. Das atlas-blockeirungs-syndrome des sauglings und des kleinkindes. Manuelle Medizin 1987;25:5–10.

33. Lewit, K. Manuelle medizin im rhamen der medizinishcen rehabilitation. Munchen, Germany: Urban & Schwartzenberg, 1977.

34. Lewit, K. Kopfgelenkblockierungen und chronische tonsillitis. Manuelle Medizin 1976;14:106–9.

35. Gutmann, G. Das atlas-blockeirungs-syndrome des sauglings und des kleinkindes. Manuelle Medizin 1987;25:5–10.

36. van Breda, WM, van Breda, JM. A comparative study of the health status of children raised under the health care models of chiropractic and allopathic medicine. J Chir Res 1989(Summer):101–3.

37. Phillips, CJ. Personal communication of prepublication report, 1992.

38. Bianchi, M, et al. Traditional acupuncture increases the content of beta-endorphin in immune cells and influences mitogen induced proliferation. Am J Chinese Med 1991;19(2):101–4.

Chapter 10: Common Conditions for Which Antibiotics are Prescribed: What You Can Do

1. Ayres, S, Mihan, R. Acne vulgaris: therapy directed at pathophysiologic defects. Cutis 1981;28:41–2.

2. Werbach, MR. Nutritional influences on mental illness. Tarzana, CA: Third Line Press, Inc., 1991:267.

3. Lidefelt, KJ, Bollgren, I, Nord, CE. Changes in periurethral microflora after antimicrobial drugs. Arch Dis Child 1991;66:683–5.

4. Ofek, I, Goldhar, J, et al. Anti-*Escherichia coli* adhesion activity of cranberry and blueberry juices. N Engl J Med

References

1991;324(22):1599.

5. Reid, G, et al. Vaginal flora and urinary tract infections. Current opinion in Infectious Disease. 1991;4:37–41.

6. Schnaubelt, K. San Rafael, CA. Personal communication, 1992.

7. Hussey, GD, Klein, M. A randomized, controlled trial of vitamin A in children with severe measles. N Engl J Med 1990;323:160–164.

8. Pinnock, CB, Douglas, RM, Badcock, NR. Vitamin A status in children who are prone to respiratory tract infections. Aust Paediatr J 1986 22:95–99.

9. Common colds: finally getting their due. Medical World News 1991;April:29:24–30.

10. Medical World News:24–30.

11. Wolfe, SM. Antibiotics. Health Letter. Washington, DC: The Public Citizen Health Research Group, 1989;5(7):1–5.

12. Pechere, JC, et al. Infections: recognition, understanding, treatment, Philadelphia: Lea & Febiger, 1984.

13. Al-Nakib, W, et al. Prophylaxis and treatment of rhinovirus colds with zinc gluconate lozenges. J Antimicrob Chemother 1987;20:893–901.

14. Medical World News:24–30.

15. Froom, J, Culpepper, L, et al. Diagnosis and antibiotic treatment of acute otitis media: report from the International Primary Care Network. Br Med J 1990;300:582–6.

16. Cantekin, EI, McGuire, TW, Griffith, TL. Antimicrobial therapy for otitis media (secretory otitis media). JAMA 1991;266(23):3309–3317.

17. Chaput de Saintonge, DM, Levine, DF. Trial of three-day and ten-day courses of amoxycillin in otitis media. Br Med J 1982;284:1078–1081.

18. Bain, J, Murphy, E, Ross, F. Acute otitis media: clinical course among children who received a short course of high-dose antibiotic. Br Med J 1985;291:1243–1246.

References

19. Hendrickse, WA, Kusmiesz, H, et al. Five vs. ten days of therapy for acute otitis media. Pediatr Inf Dis J 1988;7:14–23.

20. Meistrup-Larsen, KI, Sorenson, H, et al. Two versus seven days penicillin treatment for acute otitis media. Acta Otolaryngol 1983;96:99–104.

21. Meistrup-Larsen, et al.:99–104.

22. Klein, JO. Microbiology of otitis media. Ann Otol Rhinol Laryngol 1980;89 (Suppl 68):98.

23. Skoner, DP, Stillwagon, PK, et al. Inflammatory mediators in chronic otitis media with effusion. Arch Otolaryngol Head Neck Surg 1988;114:1131–1133.

24. Jung, TTK. Prostaglandins, leukotrienes, and other arachidonic acid metabolites in the pathogenesis of otitis media. Laryngoscope 1988;98:14–18.

25. Brown, MJ, Richards, SH, Ambegaokar, AG. Grommets and glue ear: a five-year follow-up of a controlled trial. J Roy Soc Med 1978;71:353–356.

26. Pichichero, ME, Berghash, LR, Hengerer, AS. Anatomic and audiologic sequelae after tympanostomy tube insertion or prolonged antibiotic therapy for otitis media. Ped Inf Dis J 1989;8(11):780–87.

27. Pichichero, ME. Letter, Ped Inf Dis J 1990;9(7):527–8.

28. Naunton, E. Milk sometimes culprit in ear infections: milk-free diets successful in treating ear infections. The Miami Herald 1988;Nov. 29.

29. Schmidt, MA. Childhood ear infections. Berkeley, CA: North Atlantic Books, 1990:41.

30. Doran, TF, DeAngelis, C, Baumgardner, RA, Mellitis, ED. Acetaminophen: more harm than food for chickenpox? J Pediatrics 1989;114(6):1045–8.

31. Jaffe, DM. High fever: is early antibiotic treatment useful!? N Engl J Med 1987;317:1175.

32. Hoffman, D. The holistic herbal. Moray, Scotland: Findhorn Press, 1983;112.

33. Galland, L.; Buchman, C.; Superimmunity for Kids. New York: EP Dutton, 1988;124.

34. Chow, AW, et al. Orofacial odontogenic infections. Ann Int Med 1978;88:392.

35. Rabinowitz, HK. Upper respiratory infection. In Brucker, PC, Primary care: infectious diseases. Philadelphia: WB Saunders, 1990;12:806.

36. Jones, L. Sinusitis: what you should know about your sinus problems. Springville, Utah: Madaus Murdock, 1991;4.

37. Rabinowitz, HK.:806.

38. Levin, A.; HealthFacts 1987;Jan.

39. Wang, T, Tiessen, E. Canadian Family Physician 35:1771, Sept. 1989.

40. Pichichero, ME, Disney, FA, Talpey, WB, et al. Adverse and beneficial effects of immediate treatment of group A beta-hemolytic streptococcal pharyngitis with penicillin. Ped Infect Dis J 1987;6:635–643.

41. Massel, BF, et al. N Engl J Med 1988;318:280.

42. Bisno, A. Streptococcal infections that fail to cause recurrences of rheumatic fever. J Infect Dis 1977;136:278–85.

43. Pechere, JC, et al. Infection: recognition, understanding, treatment. Philadelphia: Lea & Febiger, 1984:37.

44. Anonymous. Folk therapy for vaginitis looking good. Sci News 1992;141:158.

Index

Abuse, 172
Acne, 225–226
Acetaminophen, 46, 235.
  See also Tylenol®
Aconite, 214
Acupuncture, 218
AIDS, 145–146, 191, 203, 218
Air pollution, 120–122
  indoor, 118–120, 243
Alcohol, 82, 91, 108, 109, 145, 187, 192
Allergies, 114, 121, 133
  and antibiotics, 4
  and vitamin C, 193, 199
Allium cepa, 242
"Alternative Medicine," 265
American Dental Association, 41
American Heart Association, 41
American Journal of Chinese Medicine, 218
American Journal of Clinical Nutrition, 72, 84
American Journal of Medicine, 25
American Journal of Public Health, 119
Ames, B., 135
Amino acids, 112
Amoxicillin, 32–33, 233, 236, 243
Ampicillin, 20, 27, 227, 229
Anatomy of an Illness (Cousins), 117
Antibiotic-resistant bacteria, 9–21
  dental amalgams, 113–115
  electromagnetic fields, 116
  essential oils, 206
Anger, 174–175

Annals of the New York Academy of Sciences, 196
Antibiotics
  allergic reactions, 28–29
  and animals, 30
  attitudes about, 43–45
  and bacterial susceptibility, 30–32
  and birth control pills, 37
  broad spectrum, 23
  and chronic complaints, 25
  and chronic fatigue syndrome, 24
  dental use, 41–42
  economic costs, 29–30
  and the elderly, 33
  and fever, 48, 236
  and food allergy, 28
  hospital use, 38–40
  and immune suppression, 25–26
  infants and children, 35–36
  and infection, 15–18
  misprescribed, 4, 47–48
  and nutrient loss, 27–28
  overprescribed, 4
  parasite infection, 26–27
  physicians knowledge of, 49–51
  and pregnancy, 37
  prescriptions rise, 3–4, 35
  preventive, 5, 16, 39
  proper use, 55
  public perception, 45–46
  and recurrent infections, 25–26
  self-test, 53–54
  sinusitis, 243–244
  and stress, 158–160

teenagers, 38
tonsillitis, 246
and urinary tract infection, 5,
    226–227
and vaginal flora, 5
and vitamin C, 188, 190, 192,
    200
women's health, 37
Antibodies, 25, 63, 74, 79, 191, 207
Antifungal, 203, 204, 206, 208, 209
Apis mellifica, 214, 247
Aromatherapy.
    See essential plant oils
*Aromatherapy to Heal and Tend
    the Body* (Tisserand), 212
Arsenicum, 214
The Art of Aromatherapy
    (Tisserand), 211
Ascorbic acid. *See* vitamin C
Asfora, J., 190
Aspirin, 45–46, 77, 107–108, 192,
    235
Asthma, 120, 209

Bachmann, G.A., 172
Bacitracin, 27
Bacteria, 14, 46, 61–67
    electromagnetic fields, 116
    chiropractic, 216–217
    essential plant oils, 206–210
    herbs and, 202–204
    homeopathy and, 212–215
    stress and, 157–158
    vitamin C, 190–191, 198
Bacterial endocarditis, 18, 41–42
Barnes, B., 92
Basal Temperature Test, 92–93
Bauman, D.S., 25
Beasley, J., 40, 123, 131, 187, 188
Becker, R.O., 116–117
Belaiche, P., 208
Beliefs, 176
Belladonna, 213, 214, 234, 247, 262
Berk, L.S., 177
Beta-carotene, 98, 102, 122, 124,

128, 129, 141, 200, 228, 262
Beyond the Magic Bullet (Dixon),
    13, 70
Bifidobacterium bifidus, 22, 27, 56,
    241
Bioflavonoids, 102
Bladder infection, 3, 7, 21, 23, 36,
    37, 53, 75, 125–126, 208, 209,
    214–215, 226–229, 263
Bland, J.S., 82–83, 125
Bliznakov, E.G., 101
Block, G., 198
Blood cells, white, 6, 13, 25,
    63–68, 84–85, 99, 114, 162
    and chiropractic, 216
    and echinacea, 203
    and vitamin C, 190–192, 193
Blueberry, 53
The Body Electric (Becker), 116
The Body is the Hero (Glasser),
    201
Bonset, 236
Borneol, 208
Boyce, W.T., 156–158
Bradford, T.L., 212
Brain Allergies, 90–91
Breastfeeding, 20, 37
Breneman, J.C., 74
Brennan, P.C., 216
British Homeopathic Journal, 213
Bronchitis, 52, 75, 209, 229–230
Buchman, D.D., 95
Bulletin of the Atomic Scientist, 32
Burkitt, D., 85
Burwell, D., 3
Byrd, R., 144–145, 268

Calcium, 103, 113, 128
Calophyllum inophyllum, 242, 244
Cameron, E., 190
Campos, F.A., 72
Campylobacter, 30, 93, 238
Cancer,
    and cigarette smoke, 141
    and nutrition, 132

and vitamin C, 187, 188, 192, 197, 198

Candida albicans, 5, 7, 27, 62, 65, 109, 239, 241. *See also* Yeast
citrus seed extract and, 203
echinacea and, 203
garlic and, 203
and immune suppression, 23
thyme oil and, 207, 209
and vaginitis, 248–249

Candida-related complex (CRC), 24

Candidiasis, 208

Cantekin, E., 32–33

Cantharis, 228

Cassata, D.M., 159–160

Castleman, M., 140, 205

Cathcart, R., 190, 193, 198, 199

Cefaclor, 33, 233

Cefoxitin, 21

Centers for Disease Control (CDC), 21

Cephalexin, 28

Chamomilla, 234, 245

Chediak-Higashi disease, 132–133

Cheraskin, E., 193, 194, 197

Chickenpox, 18, 64, 72, 213, 214

Childhood Ear Infections (Schmidt), 19, 37, 76, 235

Chiropractic, 73, 216–217, 206

Cholera, 13
homeopathy and, 212, 213
Vibrio cholera, 204

Chopra, D., 178

Chronic fatigue syndrome, 73, 101, 114

Chronic Fatigue Syndrome and the Yeast Connection (Crook), 24

Cigarette smoke, 117–118, 123, 141–142, 173
and vitamin C, 187, 192

Citral, 207,

Citrus seed extract, 202

Clary sage, 234

Clindamycin, 27, 225

Clostridium dificile, 27, 34

Clove oil, 207, 248

Coenzyme Q$_{10}$, 100–101, 102

Cohen, M.L., 21

Cohen, S., 161

Cold, 3, 4, 29, 45–46, 83, 99, 119, 125, 140–141, 263
antibiotics, 231
eucalyptus, 209
garlic, 203
homeopathy, 214–215
massage, 218
selfcare, 230–232
stress, 160–161
vitamin C, 190–191, 193, 194

Cold Cures (Castleman), 140

Cold sores, 210

Comprehensive Digestive Stool Analysis, 240

Confession, 167–168, 175

Conjunctivitis, 214, 215

Coping, 89–91, 164–167, 180

Copper, 93, 102

Cortisone, 248

Cousins, N., 177

Cow's milk, 69, 75–77, 133, 232, 238, 246, 261, 264

Cranberry, 53, 227–228

Crook, W.G., 23, 24, 36, 38, 56, 75, 95

Cross Currents (Becker), 117

Crowding, 149

Cultures, 30–31, 47

Cummings, S., 215

The Cure is in the Kitchen (Rogers), 95

Cypress, 246

Cystitis. *See* Bladder infection

Dadd, D.L., 129

Dairy products. *See* Cow's milk

Day care, 149

Dentist, 40–42, 115

Depression, 114, 125, 139, 193,

195
Detoxification, 123, 262
Diarrhea, 6, 13, 34, 72, 111, 194,
 199, 238–239
Dick, E.C., 231
Diet,
 and acne, 38, 225–226
 consumption habits, 81
 and coping, 89–91
 and ear infections, 35–36
 food allergy, 74–79
Diet Prevents Polio (Sandler), 83
Diflucan, 248
Digestive enzymes, 89
Dillon, K., 177–178
Diphtheria, 15, 190
Discovering Homeopathy:
 Medicine for the 21st Century
 (Ullman), 212, 215
Disney, F.A., 49
Distemper, canine, 82, 195
Dixon, B., 13, 70, 121
Doran, T., 235
Dossey, L., 161, 164, 267–268
Down syndrome, 132
Dr. Berger's Immune Power Diet
 (Berger), 95
Drug Information, 20
Drugs, 145, 155, 187
Dyer, W., 182
Dysentery, 19, 190

E. coli, 20, 27, 203, 204, 209,
 226–227
Ear infection, 3, 6, 7, 23, 30–31,
 45, 151. *See also* otitis media
 antibiotic prescriptions and, 36
 antibiotics and recurrence, 26
 and chiropractic, 216–217
 cigarettes smoke and, 141
 cost of treatment, 29
 doctor/patient attitudes, 43–45
 duration of treatment, 29
 essential oils and, 208
 and food allergy, 75

heavy metals and, 111
 homeopathy, 214–215
 and hyperactivity, 36
 politics, 32–33
 rhinitis and, 241
 selfcare, 232–235, 261, 264
 stress and, 159–160
 teething and, 245
Echinacea, 52, 203, 236, 244, 262
Echinacea: Nature's Immune
 Enhancer (Foster), 203
Ekman, P., 175
Elderly, 33–35, 71
Electromagnetic pollution,
 115–117
Emotions, 163, 180
Encephalitis, 189, 191–192, 193
Entamoeba histolytica, 110, 204
Environment, 11, 67, 105–130, 163
Environmental illness, 29, 107,
 120–122
Environmental Protection
 Agency, (EPA), 120, 141
Environmental toxins, 67,
 107–110, 142
 dental amalgams, 113–115
 detoxification, 125
 exposure, 117–118
 heavy metals, 109, 111–113
 malnourishment, 123
 occupational, 122
 and pregnancy, 111
 protective nutrients, 112–113
 testing for, 126–127
 and vitamin C, 192
Ephedra sinica, 244
Erythromycin, 27, 72, 225
Esch, S., 205
Essential fatty acids, 73, 93
Essential plant oils, 206–212, 218
Eucalyptus, 206, 209
Eucalyptus globulus, 209, 244
Eucalyptus radiata, 209, 211, 230,
 232, 237, 244
Euphrasia, 242

Index

Evening primrose oil, 98, 103
Everybody's Guide to Homeopathic Medicines, 215
Exercise, 142–143
Expectations, 171
Eysenck, H.J., 155

Family physician, 3, 50
Fat, 84, 95–96
Fatigue, 6, 24–25, 120, 125, 139, 142, 194, 195. *See also* Chronic fatigue syndrome
Feed Your Kids Right (Smith), 37
Internal Medicine News, 39
Fever, 15, 48, 72, 111, 138, 214, 230, 235–236
Fiber, 85–87, 95
Flagyl, 248
Flax seed oil, 96, 103, 205, 234
Fleming, A., 19
Flu, 3, 46, 83, 213, 218. *See also* Influenza
Food additives, 28, 87–88, 108, 109
Food allergy (and intolerance), 74–79
 and antibiotics, 28
 causes of, 77
 common offenders, 75–76
 and ear infection, 75
 and respiratory infection, 75
 symptoms of, 77–79
 tests for, 78–79
 and tonsillitis, 75
 and toxicity, 125
Foodborne infection, 93–94
Foster, S., 203
Free radicals, 192
Frieden, T.R., 72–73

Galland, L, 24, 27, 80, 95, 239
Gard, Z., 128
Garlic, 203–204
Gattefossé, H.M., 207
Genetics, 67, 131–136

German chamomile, 236
Giardia lamblia, 7, 77, 87, 110, 204, 238
Gilbert, W., 19
Gildemeister, E., 206
Glasser, R.J., 201
D-glucaric acid, 126–127
Goldenseal, 204, 244
Gonorrhea, 18, 20–21
Gutmann, G., 216

Haemophilus influenzae, 8, 20, 21, 121, 132, 232
Hagglund, H.E., 25
Hair analysis, 113
Hands-on healing, 215
Hauser, W., 25
Hazelnut oil, 242, 244, 249
Headaches, 119, 120, 125, 126, 263
The Healing Herbs (Castleman), 205
Healthy Pleasures (Ornstein, Sobel), 152, 169, 180
Heart attack, 161
Heavy metals. *See* Environmental toxins
Helichrysum, 226, 249
Hepar sulph, 215
Hepatitis, 191, 194
Herbal medicine, 202–205
Heredity. *See* Genetics
Herpes, 210
Hoffmann, F.R., 206
Hollwich, F., 139
Holmes and Rahe, 157
Homeopathic medicine, 212–215
Hornig, D., 197
Hospital, 21, 34, 38–40
Huggins, H., 114
Human and Experimental Toxicology, 125
Hurley, L., 135
Hygiene, 136–137, 140–141
Hyperactivity, 8, 36, 90
Hypericum triquetrifolium, 52

Index

Ibuprofen, 77
Idler, E., 167
Immune system,
  and acupuncture, 218
  beta-carotene, 98
  botanical medicine, 20
  and chiropractic, 216
  and coenzyme Q$_{10}$, 100–101
  complementary treatments, 201
  description of, 61–68
  essential plant oils, 206–210,
    211
  and expectations, 171
  and homeopathy, 214
  and iron, 100
  laughter, 177–178
  and massage, 217–218
  and optimism/pessimism,
    169–170
  selenium, 100
  and social support, 172–174
  stress, 161–163
  suppression by *Candida
    albicans,* 23
  and thyroid function, 92
  and vitamin A, 97–98
  and vitamin C, 190, 192, 198
  and vitamin E, 98
  and zinc, 99–100
Immunization, 16, 189
Impetigo, 214
Infection,
  effect on nutrition, 72–73
  and vitamin C, 188–192
Infections in Medicine, 23
*Infections: Recognition,
  Understanding, Treatment*
  (Pechere), 48, 231
Infectious Disease Society of
  America, 16
Influenza, 203, 209, 214–215,
  237–238. *See also* Flu
Inner Strength®, 94, 239, 241
Interferon, 66, 204
*International Journal of Sports
  Medicine,* 143
Internist, 3, 50
Intestinal infection, 238
Inula graveolens, 206, 209, 230,
  234, 242, 244
Iron, 100, 196
Ishegami, T., 156, 170

Jaffe, D.M., 48, 236
Jaffe, R.M., 10
Jessop, C., 24
Jones, G.W., 213
Jones, L., 244
Jones, M.H., 95
*Journal of Advancement in
  Medicine,* 25
*Journal of the American Chemical
  Society,* 203
*Journal of the American Medical
  Association,* 26, 33, 189, 194,
  233
Journal of Environmental Health,
  27
Journal of Infectious Disease, 16
*Journal of the Royal Society of
  Medicine,* 75
Journaling, 181
Julius, M., 174
Justice, B., 155, 168

Kalokerinos, A., 189
Kanamycin, 27
Kasl, S., 171
Kass, E.H., 16
Keflex, 28, 29
The Kellogg Report, 123, 187
Ketoconazole, 22, 248
Kiecolt-Glaser, J., 150
Klebsiella pneumoniae, 203, 207,
  209
Klein, M.A., 198
Klenner, F., 187, 188, 193, 194,
  198, 200
Kidney stones, 196–197
Krause, R., 19

302

Krueger, J.M., 146

Lachesis, 215
Lactobacillus acidophilus, 2, 22,
  56, 66
  and B-vitamins, 22
  and bladder infections, 228
  and fever, 236
  and foodborne infection, 94
  and intestinal infections,
    238–239
  and parasites, 27
  post-antibiotic syndrome,
    240–241
  and vaginitis, 37, 249
Lancet, 8, 20, 72
Langer, S.E., 92, 134
Lappé, M., 16, 27
Laughter, 177–178
Lavender oil, 206, 207, 210, 211
Leaky gut, 22, 77
Learned Optimism (Seligman),
  170
Lemon oil, 207
Lemongrass oil, 207
Leukemia, 202
Lentinus edodes, 52, 204.
  See also Shiitake mushroom
Lewit, K., 216
Licorice root, 204
Lidefelt, K.J., 36
Life events, 156–157
Light, 138–140
Lincomycin, 27
Locke, S., 155
The Logic of Figures, 212
Lymphatic system, 162
  and chiropractic, 216–217
  and echinacea, 203
  and exercise, 142
  and massage, 217–218

McKeown, T., 11, 15–16, 71, 136
McKinlay, S.M. and J.B., 16
Macrolide, 231

Magnesium, 27, 73, 90, 103, 113,
  128, 139
Massage, 147–148, 217–218
Measles, 53, 72–73, 97, 214, 236
Medical World News, 231
Meditation, 145, 150
Melaleuca alternifolia, 245, 249.
  See also tea tree oil
Meniere's disease, 176
Meningitis, 203, 212
Meningococcus, 212
Mercapturic acid, 126, 127
Mercurius, 215, 247
Mercury amalgams, 113–115
Metchnikoff, E., 13–14
Mind, 162
Moeller, T.P., 172
Mohr, U., 216
Mold, 118, 120
Mononucleosis, 199
Moskowitz, H., 173
Mothering, 177
Mowrey, D.B., 203, 205
Mumps, 214
Mycoplasma pneumoniae, 157

National Academy of Sciences,
  117, 187
National Cancer Institute, 10, 187,
  188, 198
National Institute of Allergies and
  Infectious Diseases, 19
National Institutes of Health, 10,
  19, 32, 151
National Research Council, 186
Neisseria meningitidis, 212
Neomycin, 27, 208
Nervous system, 162
Neu, H.C., 21
Newberne, P.M., 69, 71
New England Journal of
  Medicine, 33, 44, 227
Niaouli, 211, 230
Nieman, D., 143
Noise, 148–149

Non-Toxic and Natural (Dadd), 129
The Non-Toxic Home (Dadd), 129
Novobiocin, 27
Nsouli, T.M., 75
Nutrition,
    absorption, 77
    anti-nutrients, 87–88
    and coping, 89–91
    and hospital patients, 39
    and immunity, 70–72
    and infection-susceptibility, 70–72
    physician's knowledge of, 51–52
    content of refined food, 86
Nutritional Influences in the Cause of Infectious Disease, 71
Nutritional supplementation, 96–102
Nystatin, 37, 56, 248

Obesity, 82–83
Obstetrician/gynecologist, 3, 50
Ochsner, G., 149
Omega-3 fatty acids, 96, 103
Opening Up: The Healing Power of Confiding in Others (Pennebaker), 168
Optimism, 168–171
Oregano oil, 207, 208, 247
Ornstein, R., 152, 169, 174, 180
Oscillococcinum, 213, 237
Oski, F., 77
Otitis media.
    See also Ear infections
    antibiotics as a cause, 4
    and chiropractic, 217
    and essential oils, 208
    and vitamin C, 193

Paget, J., 146
Paradox of antibiotics, 14–15
Parasites, 26–27, 77, 110
    and essential oils, 210
    and herbs, 202

and homeopathy, 213
Pasteur, L., 14
Pauling, L., 185, 186, 190, 194–195, 197, 198
Pediatricians, 3, 50, 150–151
Pediatrics, 49
Pediazole, 33, 233
Pennebaker, J.W., 167
Penicillin, 5, 14–15, 19, 20–21, 46, 188, 203, 204, 207, 227, 231
Penn, N.D., 34
Perception, 165, 166–167
Pertussis. *See* Whooping cough
Pessimism, 168–171
Pesticides, 19, 117, 187
Peterson, C., 169
Phagocytosis, 25, 63, 190, 207
Phenol, 206–207
Phillips, C.J., 217
Philpott, W., 90
Physicians,
    diagnostic accuracy, 47–48
    knowledge of antibiotics, 48–51
    knowledge of nutrition, 51–52
Physician's Desk Reference, 30–31
Placebo, 176
Plantago major, 234, 245
Please, Don't Drink Your Milk (Oski), 77
Pleasure, 152
Pneumonia, 5, 15, 18–19, 21, 34, 53, 75, 97, 120–121, 191, 229–230, 231, 237
Polymixin, 27
Porter, R.R., 15
Post-antibiotic syndrome, 239–241
Power, 172
The Practice of Aromatherapy (Valnet), 211
Prayer, 144–145
Pregnancy, 37, 80, 82, 98, 100, 111, 129, 135–136, 204, 211
    herbs to avoid, 250
Probioplex®, *See* Inner Strength®

Prontosol, 188
Prostatitis, 227
Proteus, 203, 233
Psychoneuroimmunology, 180
Pullen, F., 76, 234
Pulsatilla, 234
Pyrogen, 213
Ravensare aromatica, 233, 237
Recovering the Soul (Dossey), 267
Red meat, 95
Relationships, 172–174
Relaxation, 150
Remington, J., 25
Respiratory infection, 21, 36, 52,
    72, 75, 120–122, 140–141
    and echinacea, 203
    and eucalyptus, 209
    and stress, 156–159
    and thyme, 209
Rheumatic fever, 15, 247
Rhinitis, 241–243
Rhus tox, 213, 214
Ringsdorf, W.M., 197
Rivers, J.M., 196
Roberts, D.W., 105
Rogers, S., 95, 117
The Role of Medicine
    (McKeown), 136
Rommelt, H., 207
Rosa rubiginosa, 211
Rosemary officinalis (verbinone),
    230, 242, 244, 249
Rowe, A., 78

Saccharin, 28
Sachs, B.C., 155
Salmonella, 30, 93, 203, 238
Salmonella newport, 8–9
Sandler, B., 83
Sauna, 127–128, 137–138, 264
Savory oil, 208, 211, 247
Schmidt, Michael A., 19, 37, 69,
    75, 76, 138, 178, 235
Schnaubelt, K., 207, 208
Science, 19, 21

*The Scientific Validation of Herbal
    Medicine* (Mowbrey), 203, 205
Scurvy, 185, 186, 194, 196
Seasonal affective disorder
    (SAD), 139
Sehnert, K.W., 52, 138, 223
Selenium, 100, 102, 112, 113, 122,
    124, 128, 129, 262
Seligman, M., 169–170
Selye, H., 155, 158
Shigella, 241
Shiitake mushroom, 204
Sick building syndrome, 118–120
Silymarin, 129
Sinus, 3, 45, 83, 141, 209, 217,
    243–244, 262
Skoner, D.P., 31
Sleep, 146–147, 187
Smith, L.H., 37, 90, 191
Sobel, D., 152, 169, 174, 180
Solomon, G., 180
Solved: The Riddle of Illness
    (Langer), 92
Sore throat, 3, 47, 111, 121,
    214–215, 246–248, 262.
    See also Tonsillitis
Space, Time and Medicine
    (Dossey), 267
Spectinomycin, 21
Speirs, R.S., 105
Staph, 19, 27, 190, 203, 204
Staphylococcus aureus, 27, 110,
    204, 207
Stitt, P.A., 84
Strep, 9, 18, 19, 27, 47, 203, 204,
    246, 262
Streptococci, 27, 57, 158
Streptococcus pneumoniae, 21,
    132, 232
Streptococcus viridans, 110
Streptomycin, 204, 207
Stress, 67
    and common cold, 160–161
    and coping, 164–167
    and immunity, 161–163

and infection susceptibility,
155–160
and laughter, 177
and massage, 217
and vitamin C, 186, 187
Sucrose, 28
Sugar, 83–85, 91, 95
Sulfonamide, 7, 14–15, 25
Superimmunity for Kids
(Galland), 80, 95
Supplements. *See* Nutritional
supplementation
Support, 172–174
Surgeons, 50
Susceptibility testing, 30–32
Syphilis, 18

Tagamet, 124
Tea tree oil, 53, 207, 208, 211, 228,
236, 245, 263. *See also*
Melaleuca alternifolia
Teething, 245–246
Television, 89, 142
Tetanus, 190
Tetracycline, 25, 37, 38, 72, 225,
229, 231
Thyme oil, 207, 208–209, 247–248
Thymus, 97, 101, 162, 163
Thymus vulgaris.
See also Thyme oil
thuyanol (CT), 209
thymol (CT), 249
Thyroid dysfunction, 91–93,
133–134
Tierra, M., 205
Time, 265
Tisserand, R., 148, 209, 211, 212
Toluene, 123, 125
Tonsillitis, 4, 6, 7, 9–10, 30, 48, 49,
52, 69, 72, 83, 97, 119, 133, 157,
203. *See also* Sore throat
and chiropractic, 216–217
and massage, 218
selfcare, 246–248
Touch, 147–148, 215

Trans fatty acids, 96, 103
Trimethoprim-sulfamethoxazole,
25, 227, 229
Tschetter, D., 42
Tuberculosis, 16, 19, 156, 170, 190,
204
Tylenol®, 235
Type A personality, 164–165
Type B personality, 165
Typhoid, 190

Udintsev, Y.N., 116
Ullman, D., 212, 215
UltraClear®, 83, 126

Vaginal infection, 125–126, 23, 30,
38
selfcare, 248–249
and tea tree oil, 208
and thyme oil, 209
van Breda, W. and J., 150, 217
Victims, 164, 179–180
Viruses, 4, 9, 26, 29, 36, 45–46,
61–67, 140
cold, 231
Epstein-Barr, 73, 171
and essential oils, 206–209
and herbs, 202–204
and homeopathy, 213–215
influenza, 237
RSV, 242
and stress, 157–158
and vitamin C, 190–191, 198
Vitamin C, 34, 40, 52, 71, 73, 93,
98, 102, 112–113, 122, 123, 124,
128, 129, 135, 136, 141
and bladder infection, 228
and bronchitis, 230
and cancer, 187
different needs for, 186–187
dosage of, 193–194
and infectious disease, 188–192,
231–237
and rhinitis, 242
RDA, 186

rules for use, 198–200
safety, 196–197
and scurvy, 185–186
signs of deficiency, 195
and stress, 186
and tetracycline, 72
and vaginitis, 249
The Vitamin C Connection
(Cheraskin), 197
Vitamins,
A, 34, 53, 71, 72–73, 80, 93, 97,
101, 123, 124, 226, 228, 229,
230, 249
B-complex, 112, 128, 262
B₂, 93
B₃, 93
B₅, 102
B₆, 93, 102, 123, 226
B₁₂, 95, 196, 226
D, 139
E, 34, 71, 93, 98, 101, 112, 123,
124, 128, 129, 141, 200, 226,
249
von Pettenkofer, M., 13

Walnut oil, 208
Walsh, J., 146

The Way of Herbs (Tierra), 205
Welch, G.H., 20
Weatherford, J., 137
Weinstein, L., 16
Werbach, M.R., 80
When Antibiotics Fail (Lappé), 27
Witkin, S.S., 23
Who Gets Sick (Justice), 155, 168
Whooping cough, 15, 52, 189, 203
Williams, G., 69, 71
Williams, R., 134, 174–175, 187,
199
World Health Organization, 61, 69

Yarrow, 236
The Yeast Connection (Crook), 22
The Yeast Connection Cookbook
(Crook, Jones), 95
Yeast, 5, 31, 36, 37
description of, 46
vaginal, 23, 30, 38
Yellow fever, 212
Yogurt, 249

Zinc, 27–28, 71, 72, 80, 93,
99–100, 113, 123, 14, 128, 129,
135, 225, 231, 249, 261

About the Authors

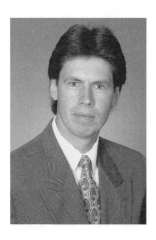

Dr. Michael A. Schmidt is an author, lecturer and researcher in preventive health care. He is author of *Childhood Ear Infections: What Every Parent and Physician Should Know,* which was called "a true jewel" by *Holistic Medicine.* Co-author of *Managing the Patient with Chronic Fatigue,* he edits *Current Topics in Preventive Pediatrics and Family Practice.* A former analytical chemist and technical assistant in microbiology, Dr. Schmidt began a nutrition-oriented private practice in 1983 in Anoka, Minnesota.

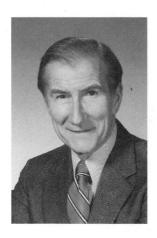

Dr. Lendon H. Smith is a humorist and internationally renowned pediatrician, author and lecturer. He has written over ten books on health and nutrition and is one of the pioneers of preventive medicine. His best known books are *Feed Your Kids Right* and *Feed Yourself Right.* Known as "The Childrens' Doctor," he has been a frequent guest on "Phil Donahue," "The Tonight Show" and "Oprah Winfrey." His syndicated "TV Health Tips" has aired since 1977.

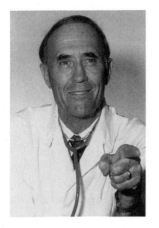

Dr. Keith W. Sehnert, author of *Stress/ Unstress, Selfcare/Wellcare* and *How to Be Your Own Doctor (Sometimes),* has brought medical self-care as a popular concept to a large audience. His work has been featured in *Family Health, Parade, Newsweek, Ladies Home Journal, Mc- Calls, Money* and *Reader's Digest.* Dr. Sehnert is in private practice in Min- neapolis, Minnesota.

Author Correspondence

Dr. Michael A. Schmidt
P.O. Box 452
Anoka, MN 55303

Dr. Lendon H. Smith
P.O.Box 427
Portland, OR 97207

Dr. Keith W. Sehnert
4210 Freemont Ave. S.
Minneapolis, MN 55409